Dear Jill,

To my good FRIEND &
Birthday group partner.
To our good health FROM
GOD's Bountiful garden.
Love you.

Karen

No Diagnosis

by

Karen Ament

ISBN 978-0-9903935-3-5

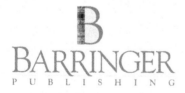

BARRINGER
P U B L I S H I N G

Table of Contents

Introduction

"I have been driven many times to my knees by the overwhelming conviction that I had nowhere else to go."   Abraham Lincoln

I HAD ALWAYS BEEN A PRAYERFUL person who realized from an early age that God was in charge of my life. He died for my sins, and I was His child. He had saved me, and for this I was deeply appreciative. But I had not been driven to my knees as Abraham Lincoln was until a strange malady took over my healthy body and changed my normal days into days of confusion, pain, and fear. As a trained registered nurse, I knew there were unusual illnesses, but I also knew that the medical community could analyze and test for even the most unusual cases and come to some logical conclusion. They were not afraid of tackling any and every symptom to categorize and diagnose most diseases, and I also knew that, if they were in doubt, they would move heaven and earth to get to the bottom of every case presented to them.

Or at least I used to know this . . .

At first when my initial symptoms surfaced, I just assumed while there was some embarrassment as to the strangeness of my story and symptoms, it would be quickly resolved with a simple blood or stool test and prescription medications would soon relieve it. I had all the confidence in the world that this would be the case. When my symptoms emerged, I only had a gynecologist, Dr. F. My visits were usually yearly and required very little follow up. I had no diseases and was on no medication. I was through menopause and was doing well with no complaints. I was happy and content with my marriage to Bob and so proud of our children. They were college grads and on their way to successful lives and careers. I enjoyed our business and was grateful that all four of our parents were alive and doing well.

I had total confidence in all doctor opinions and would never consider taking or doing anything not medically approved. In short, I was an extremely healthy person and a compliant patient.

Until July, 1996. My confidence in the medical community would go from total to almost non-existent in a period of less than a year. Never during this time did I feel any doctor purposely ignored me or didn't try to help me. Maybe it would have spurred me on to step outside the medical box sooner if that had been the case. After all, our good medical doctors were utilizing the talents and skills they had been taught in medical school. They knew a lot. They had seen a lot. They diagnosed illnesses based on logical conclusions and on data they were familiar with. There were established parameters that could be used over and over.

After I was well and perused the doctor notes, I was surprised to see that my dermatologist, OB/Gyn, and internist felt I met the criteria for consideration of D.P. (delusional parasitosis) as nothing else seemed to fit. I was alarmed that I had fallen into a black hole of sorts. Even though I had developed systemic symptoms and was becoming very ill, because my initial complaint was unexplainable medically, and I referred to bug bites—D.P. seemed logical. This narrow scope did not leave any room to look outside the box. I can understand now that conventional medicine has to work this way in order to facilitate in an orderly fashion the process from initial complaint to treating the symptoms that develop later one by one.

However logical this process is, I have become acutely aware that many thousands of people are inadvertently falling through the cracks. They do not have D.P., and even though they meet one or two of the criteria's for D.P., they by no means meet all the criteria. Also their physical symptoms are a complete mystery and somehow are not included for consideration when they start to develop life threatening illnesses.

The doctors treat them for those but never rescind their original diagnosis of D.P. Many of these people are put on medications for mental illness and consequently can never escape the stigma from this first diagnosis. Worse yet the prescribed medications do nothing to cure the patient and are nothing more than a band aid with side effects. These side effects can sometimes compound. On top of their original symptoms, they now have added a new set of side effects caused by their being medicated. A vicious cycle has now been set in motion, and escape is nearly impossible from this prison brought on by care and concern for the patient by the caregiver completely oblivious to the damage being wrought by themselves.

Paula J. Caplan, a clinical and research psychologist is a fellow in the Women in Public Policy Program at Harvard's Kennedy School of Government. She is the author of "They say you're crazy; How the World's Most Powerful Psychiatrists decide who's normal."

In a column for the *Washington Post,* she states, "About half of all Americans get a psychiatric diagnosis in their lifetimes. Receiving any of the 374 psychiatric labels—from nicotine dependence disorder to schizophrenia—can cost anyone their health insurance, job, custody of their children, or right to make their own medical and legal decisions. And if patients take psychiatric drugs, they risk developing physical disorders such as diabetes, heart problems, weight gain, and other serious conditions. In light of the subjectivity of these diagnoses and the harm they can cause, we should be extremely skeptical of them."

But God was not content with my contentment. He had plans for me that put me out of my comfort zone and finally sent me to my knees with the overwhelming conviction that I had nowhere else to go. This is my story of survival fighting an unnamed illness with God's ever-present love. The edges of my life have been polished and rounded. I thank God daily for leading me out of that valley of darkness I found myself in from July 1996 to 2001. I now love normal days and consider each day a gift from God to be cherished. During the more than five years that I fought this thing I decided to compartmentalize my days.

To my family, friends, business associates, and customers I was my normal self. In reality I was a very sick person getting sicker and sicker with no help from my previously trusted medical community. Only my husband, Bob, could get a glimpse of the blackness, exhaustion, exasperation and fear. To fight a battle on two fronts took all the energy I could muster. One front was to overcome my disease, and the other dealt with the fact that there would be no help for me from the medical community. With no diagnosis there would be no treatment.

The summer of 1996 seems so very far away.

It is now twenty-one years later, and I have been well for the last sixteen. Could this all have been part of a bad dream? I have shared with some family and friends bits and pieces of the ordeal but not to any great extent. Mostly, I have shared trying to explain what worked for me to get well in hopes that they themselves might utilize some of the same methods to get well from an ailment they were fighting. But what I finally realized was that each person must arrive at the spot in their own lives when they have an overwhelming conviction that they have nowhere else to go. If they are not there yet, any advice, however well-meaning, will fall on deaf ears. So I am content I don't have to go back there. Why bring up an unpleasant period that is old news? For twenty-one years I did just that.

A few years ago, I was checking e-mails and the usual flurry of back and forth between family and friends. Suddenly I had an impulse to check out the status of a mysterious illness that had similar symptoms to my own. Several years before, I gathered as much information as possible on this illness and corresponded with a few sufferers and then dropped the ball. I really didn't want to be associated in any way with these poor people, and my experience trying to help others was not going very well, so no news was good news. End of story. Or at least I thought.

I typed in to my Google search bar "MORGELLONS" Up came the usual data I had seen several years earlier. Morgellons sufferers have symptoms so bizarre and baffling they defy description, but they are eerily close to my own so many years ago. After reading through testimonials and the web page for the Morgellons Foundation, I was horrified to read that no cure was yet to be found. The CDC was still studying the disease. The sufferers were still suffering, and the medical community still seemed baffled or worse, still in denial that these people (including children) had anything at all except "delusional parasitosis." I shivered with dread and such overwhelming sadness that so many were still suffering but worse—with no diagnosis.

After all my symptoms from 1996 to 2001 were gone and my box of notes and pleadings and constant searching for help and medical records were in a dusty box labeled: BOOK INFO-DO WHEN TIME. This is a note that really means PROBABLY NEVER. My box would probably be discarded someday when our kids cleaned out our home while we moved on to an assisted-living apartment or were no longer on this Earth. I had come to love my normal and knew that to open a can of worms and make this period of my life so public was not something I relished. To write a book, then actually publish it and try to market it and probably lose money on it, not to mention identify with a disease that doctors and the public still would think of as delusional, had not been high on my list.

But if there was even a slim possibility that a researcher, medical doctor or the CDC (Center for Disease Control) would see this book and something would click so the pieces of my puzzle would fit into place and, voila, an answer, diagnosis, and even a cure would emerge for so many suffering people, I absolutely had no other choice. "Why me Lord?" did cross my mind many times. But then I thought, "Why not me Lord?"

"Be on your guard! Make certain that you do not forget, as long as you live, what you have seen with your own eyes. Tell your children and grandchildren." Deuteronomy 4:9 Good News Bible

Now the testimonials I read with all the anguish, despair, anger, and hopelessness all came crashing into my normal. Surely I should not have to feel responsible to share data and experiences I had almost long forgotten. But it appeared people were still suffering, and a cure was not to be had. Perhaps a clue might lie within my notes and research accumulated from 1996 to 2001. I was one of those tortured souls. My story lay mostly within the confines of a box very dusty by now. Because you're reading this now, you know my Pandora's Box was opened. I thank God for the spirituality and calm acceptance of life's twists and turns and my healing so many years ago. But did He give me this challenge to soldier through it, amass a ton of data and then bury it in a box? Instinctively I knew what the answer was and a song from my childhood popped into my head that I used to hear my dad sing often—He was a World War II vet. "Here we go over the wild blue yonder off with one hell of a roar, to live and die to fight and fly, I'm in the Army Air Corps." This song never seemed to apply to me personally, but I always thought it pushed people to limits they never thought possible. I guess this is where I am now.

PART I

INFECTED BY SOMETHING.
Why Am I So Sick?

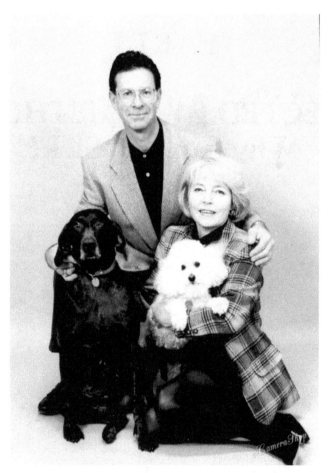

Karen Ament and her husband, Bob, were empty-nesters in 1996 with three grown children and two enjoyable dogs, Brit (German Shorthair), and Lacey, (Bichon).

Chapter One

Infected by Something

T HE YEAR 1996 HELD THE PROMISE to be a remarkable year. My husband, Bob, and I were co-owners of a successful swimming pool and spa business with two locations. We had established the business in 1971. Business was booming. During our high season we had ten to fifteen employees. We were empty nesters with two dogs—Lacey, a Bichon, and Brit, a German shorthair—to keep us company as our three children were grown.

Bob and I were learning to play golf in anticipation of our future retirement. We had a wonderful family, friends, and lots of social activities to attend. Our three children were all doing well. Our youngest son was already happily married to his high-school sweetheart. Our sons were partners at a financial services company. Their business was growing. Our only daughter had recently graduated as a registered nurse and had just gotten married on June 1st. There had been the usual hustle and bustle planning and organizing the wedding. The wedding was perfect—beautiful bride, handsome groom, and happy family and friends. All four of our parents were present. We all danced the night away, and I never felt better.

After the wedding it was back to work for Bob and me as it was our busiest season. However, our hunting dog, Brit, had torn a cruciate ligament while hunting with Bob early in the spring, and it was not healing. Our local vet suggested the best place to repair her injury was the University of Minnesota Veterinarian Teaching Hospital with the surgeon: Dr. A.L.

Brit was admitted July 15th, 1996, and discharged July 17th, coming home with Butorphanol and Torbutol for pain. When we entered the building to pick her up, I noticed it was not the usual veterinarian's office. I saw assorted animals in the cages, not the typical dogs and cats I would have expected. I remember being curious and asked why they were there. The receptionist said simply, "For research." I thought that was odd but dismissed it and took Brit home. (I phone interviewed Dr. A.L. recently, and his memory is that the animals I had seen were only dogs and cats. He made no comment on any research done there.)

Shortly after we picked up Brit, Bob and I and our two dogs went to our cabin to relax. We noticed that Brit seemed to be urgently scratching at herself and was disturbed. We assumed it was fleas she picked up at the university, so we purchased bug bombs and set them off in the cabin. We flea dipped her and Lacey. That night we all slept in our gazebo to avoid the fumes.

To our astonishment, the next day Brit was still scratching and our little Bichon Lacey was doing the same. Even worse, Bob and I experienced severe itching and a crawling sensation.

This was the beginning. Bob's symptoms were relatively short lived, lasting only a few weeks. I wasn't so lucky. Little did I know that it would be more than five years before I would feel normal again. This "thing," whatever it was, would take over my conscious and unconscious thoughts. I was uncomfortable. I became obsessed with finding a cure.

My mind raced with finding out what this itching was, and what I need to do to get rid of it. Understand that the itching was tremendously intense and, for me, localized along my torso and the fronts of my legs, eventually migrating to the back of my head, which became a focal point with drilling pain that I could not ignore. Many other symptoms were added as I became systemically ill!

What started as a simple annoyance to be dealt with by determination and resourcefulness on a private basis turned into an embarrassing series of public revelations to doctors. I was determined to stay as normal as possible while fighting this thing, but it did get nearly impossible to do so.

My washing machine was going non-stop as I washed absolutely everything I could, first at the cabin where everything else was scrubbed from top to bottom and then again at our home. I washed our bedding often as well as our dogs bedding, and the dogs got frequent baths. Usually days went pretty well while at work, but the constant zipping and zapping and drilling sensations plus itching made it very interesting at times, very distracting. I would be doing a sales presentation in the middle of a particularly wild attack and, of course, I did not want to scratch myself or show the emotional state an attack caused. I practiced looking cool, calm and collected. There was no point in doing otherwise.

Looking back, I wonder if I should have gone to a doctor sooner, maybe the emergency room to start with. I did make an appointment with my clinic several days after I was infected but was not able to see the doctor until several weeks later. I never believed this would go on so long or that I would get so ill. I felt I would lick this in a short time. Bob had.

I showered three to four times a day and often in the middle of the night. I also scrubbed the dogs a lot as they were still scratching and acting disturbed. From a calm, resting position, suddenly they would snap at a part of their bodies and chew on it.

When I finally collapsed into bed, I slept soundly for a couple of hours. Then the dreaded stuff would start to move. It would wake me up with a vengeance, so I would shower, rub lotions on the areas affected and then go down to spend the rest of the night on the couch. There was no sense keeping Bob awake all night with me. If I got four hours of sleep a night during this period, I was lucky. I kept thinking with all the cleanliness routines whatever I had would soon dissipate. I used flea scrubs on both the dogs and even myself, also chlorine along with Therapeutic T/Gel shampoo for possible psoriasis. My appetite decreased as I was totally preoccupied with my situation. I started to feel physically sick with numerous body aches, and my glands were sore. I began to have difficulty climbing stairs and needed to stop and grab onto the railing. I was becoming an invalid.

What a waste of time all this was! While I was scrubbing on an external basis, internally something was raging through my body. Late at night when I could not sleep, I spent hours and hours on the internet trying to search out what this could possibly be. Nothing connected or made sense. I knew I was treading on thin ice and moving outside the establishment thinking when I felt obligated to consider the myriad of symptoms, including the impossible ones. I came to believe that to discount what was actually happening in order to fit into an established pattern of a particular illness would not get me well. Perhaps my strange initial symptoms and subsequent systemic illness might trigger a researcher to connect the dots.

Is it mandatory to always use established data to evaluate all illnesses? Are some common but impossible modern illnesses somehow linked to these black holes at the edge of science? Is a cure for them linked in any way? I knew I needed to be honest and report all data as I lived it no matter how embarrassing it was, so here goes . . .

Chapter Two

Initial Visits to Doctors

FTER SEVERAL WEEKS OF THIS MADNESS, I started to notice small black spots on the white tile in the bathroom and shower. Also black spots were on our dogs' bedding. Then I noticed black spots on my skin, primarily on my abdomen and upper torso. When I brushed them off a small blood spot would remain. But all of this was nothing compared to what was to come. I began to notice tiny flying insects in the shower and bathroom. My senses told me they were harmless and must be coming in from outside. I sprayed with insect spray inside and outside of our home and especially profusely in our shower area.

More and more of these insects accumulated, forcing me to frequently scrub our bath and shower areas with chlorine. These same insects would fly around our dogs, and sometimes I felt them around me. I even observed them in the bath tub while I was bathing, especially when I added a little chlorine to the water. I finally had to consider the impossible possibility that they were coming from the black spots I found on my body and on the tile in the bathroom.

I decided to capture several of them in a jar and take them to St. Cloud State University and ask the biology department to identify them. I thought surely this would give me the information I needed to solve this mystery. But no luck. The biology expert said they were fungus gnats and harmless. How in the world was I going to explain this to a doctor? How could I even explain this to myself? Why would anyone believe some harmless fungus gnat was causing me such intense syptoms and my growing illness?

This was all totally unbelievable. If I weren't in the middle of it, I was sure I would never have believed anyone who told me any of this nonsense. But it was absolutely real . . . and it was happening to me. It was time to tell someone about it. I simply had no other choice.

On August 14, 1996, I had my first visit to see Dr. L. a St. Cloud internal medicine specialist. This was the beginning of an intense five years of my life dealing with the medical community. At that visit, my vital signs were normal.

"Patient comes in with what she calls an 'unusual disease.'" wrote the doctor. "Within the last month her dog was at the University of Minnesota hospitals and, while there, she thinks the dog came down with some type of unusual parasite. Subsequently, her other dog came down with 'fleas' as well, and they have been dipped four to five times apiece. Subsequently, she started breaking out in lesions on her torso, groin, and arms. She says she will get a tiny crusting on her skin and subsequently a parasite will actually hatch from the skin and turn into a bug. She has self-treated with chlorine. She says that a couple of days ago her glands were sore and she ached all over, but she doesn't know of any definite fever or chills. After she rinsed with chlorine, she was checking her hair and these bugs started to fly over her hair. She combed her hair out and has four to five bugs which she brings in a jar now. The only thing I can see is a single pustular area on the right forearm. I took a scraping but did not see anything other than skin on the scraping. Cardiac exam is normal. Lungs are clear. Abdomen is soft and nontender. No organomegaly or masses. Bones and joints appear to be normal. CBC and sedimentation rate are both normal also. I called dermatologist Dr. E., who will see her today with regard to this and do a skin scraping or punch biopsy of the lesion on her skin.

"IMPRESSION: 1. Possible fleas or unusual parasitic infestation.

"Dermatologic referral is done. Dr. E. will actually see her today."

That same day I had an appointment with the dermatologist Dr. E., and it was an uneventful visit. I was prescribed a sulfa cream. I was hoping he would be able to tell what I had just by looking at me and hearing my story but no such luck.

"Try and learn what pleases the Lord. Have nothing to do with the worthless things that people do, things that belong to the darkness."
Eph. 5:10-11 *Good News Bible*

These last three weeks have involved a lot of darkness. My nights were simply tortuous. I filled my days with survival tactics to be normal while fighting this unknown entity. I turned to God in prayer as often as I could, but mostly all I could say was simply, "Jesus, help me." I hoped someday sense could be made out of this, but I also knew this might be a long way off. I determined to fight this evil by refusing to co-operate with it. This would be easier said than done.

Yes, this illness was unusual, to say the least. Dr. L. did listen carefully. I felt I had to be honest and report exactly what was happening. I carefully looking at his face when I was telling him my ridiculous assumptions, watching for any sense of disbelief. I was sure he would consider I had lost it. I dreaded having to explain the symptoms I was having. But I felt, to get to the bottom of this strange disease, I had to be totally honest. My doctor would then remember something in an infectious disease medical book that he could point to and say, "That's it, and it's very rare, and this is what we'll have to do to treat you. It will be over soon."

Whew! Was that a Wizard of Oz thought! But he held his stoic demeanor and seemed genuinely to want to help me. But there was no mention of a possibility of a diagnosis. On rereading his notes, I couldn't help but wonder what his actual thoughts were regarding the "bugs" I talked about. Only crazy people talk about "bugs." He patiently waited me out as I described the last four weeks of agony. I did spare some of the details so as not to appear totally obsessed or, worse, demented.

I went back to work after my two doctor appointments and tried to catch up—bank deposits, daily income totals were behind, payroll needed to be done, employee schedules had to be made, inventory needed to be ordered, return calls must be made, advertising deadlines—plus it was our busy season. Many customers needed help and advice, and I gave many sales presentations. Life went on.

I washed my hands frequently and used hand sanitizer until my hands were red and raw. I was starting to be concerned I might be contagious even though both doctors said I was not. I was encouraged when it became clear that no one with whom I'd had contact ever exhibited the symptoms I had. This was a huge relief, but I was still very conscious of the possible contagion factor.

After work one day, we had dinner with some of our neighborhood friends. We enjoyed busy chatter about our families, exchanged pictures, and everyone had a good time. I made no mention of my situation and secret dilemma. What could I possibly say? My symptoms continued throughout the evening. Of course I ignored them. I also hated to leave our gathering and go home to the hellish night I knew I would face again.

The sulfa cream the dermatologist prescribed for me did not help. However it seemed to give me a little better sleep for a few more hours. I used up the tube quickly.

"Be determined and confident. Do not be afraid. Your God the Lord himself will be with you. He will not fail you or abandon you."

Deut. 31:6 Good News Bible

NURSE NOTES
REASON: The patient calls in after having an office visit two days ago for possible parasite. Was referred to dermatology and they prescribed sulfa cream which helped but did not cure her problem. She is requesting to have her stools tested for parasites. She has a specimen.
REVIEWED WITH: Dr. M.

RESPONSE: Go ahead and run ova and parasite x1. Request stool sample at the lab. (08/20/96).

All tests were negative so here I was back to square one. Tortured nights ran into difficult days. I hardly slept. The constant itching and crawling and biting and stinging were much worse at night. Sitting up and reading (researching, actually) kept my mind off of "it" for a while, but it was very hard to ignore.

I had a busy day at work. I also was packing and shopping as our family was joining us at our cabin for the weekend. While looking forward to the company, I was frantic that I was possibly contagious. I planned to use sterile techniques while handling any food items but felt nervous about contagion. It also would be difficult to be up most of the night in a small cabin with other people around.

My thought for the day: An admission of error is a sign of strength rather than a weakness. Father, give me the courage to admit when I am wrong and then to go on living in your freedom.

I took comfort in this thought all day. I had to see this illness as a way to find strength and never forget that God would not fail me and would remain with me throughout whatever was to come.

Chapter Three

First Treatments

O N August 30, 1996, I had another appointment with the dermatologist, Dr. S. His notes read: "This is a fifty-four-year-old female who is seen for a strange story that begins approximately the 16th of July at which time one of her dogs had surgery at the University. Subsequent to bringing that dog back home, apparently the dog did a lot of scratching and eventually was treated by the vet for the possibility of parasites. Shortly thereafter this patient began experiencing what she describes as 'severe symptoms' consisting of brief periods of intense itching, a 'fluttering' sensation, which will occur in the face, and a sensation of 'bites,' which will feel like a mosquito bite happening at scattered places multiple times during the day. None of these things lasts more than just a few seconds. She has been developing what she says are spots on her skin for which she needs a magnifying glass to see them. These sensations have not responded to multiple topical things that she has tried and she has seen a dermatologist who apparently did not find any abnormality. She comes in now thinking that she has a parasite, and she has treated herself for lice with over-the-counter medications without improvement.

"Examination shows no real rash. There are multiple pinpoint one millimeter or smaller lesions on the anterior thigh and several on the abdomen, which appear sub-epithelial. They are slightly red but are non-blanching. Scraping done, which failed to exhibit any nits or signs of scabies. There is no involvement of the webs of the fingers.

"I have very little to offer her. I really don't have any idea what this is. The only thing I can come up with is the possibility that she did have some scabies infestation and just a lot of superimposed itching and somatization related to that. Therefore, I have decided to try her on some Periactin for symptomatic relief of the itching and gave her a course of Kwell Shampoo and Lotion and to be seen back PRN."

On September 4th, I call the doctor's office.

NURSE NOTES: REASON: "Prescription for Periactin 4 mg one every six hours prn count of 20 was called to Walmart Pharmacy along with the Kwell Shampoo 2 oz. and Kwell Lotion 4 oz. to use as directed.

I wasn't getting relief. I had worked all week designing and laying out our fall sales flyer. We send out approximately 4,500 flyers every spring and fall to notify customers of specials. I worked through the itching and crawling and biting and stinging, and I try hard to ignore it all. I felt like Dr. Jekyll and Mr. Hyde.

Perhaps at the Last Day all that will remain worth recording of a life full of activity and zeal, will be those little deeds done solely beneath the eye of God. *Lord, help me to remember that the smallest job done in your name is very worthwhile. Teach me to rejoice in whatever task is set before me.*

I had had a hard night and faced a busy day at work and a doctor's appointment with dermatologist Dr. S. I had hoped he would get to the bottom of this illness. But instead, for the first time, I was hit hard with the word "somatization," "a mental disorder characterized by recurring multiple and current clinically significant complaints about somatic symptoms." En.m.Wikipedia.org

Neither the Kwell Shampoo nor lotion helped me long term. I did get relief initially, but it was a short-term blessing.

But for today, I decided to continue to perform acts of kindness and generosity to those around me. I would be cheerful and concerned about other people and not just worry about me.

I dropped off the flyer layout at the printer. Our whole staff will work hard next week folding, stapling and putting addresses on these flyers. We are training a new manager at our second location in Willmar (a small town sixty miles from our St. Cloud main store). It's a very busy time for us.

At the same time I was trying to keep up with my normal life, I had to deal with my not-so-normal sick life: My symptoms are changing to include my face and eye area and really strong head involvement. The face involvement distracts me immensely. Visually, I can observe little twitches, little zips and tingles streak across my face, head, scalp, nose, and eye area. I am starting to notice considerably more joint pain.

NURSE NOTES: From dermatologist office. REASON: "Pt. called on September 3rd, stating that she had huge relief with the Kwell but she has noticed that there is a tracking on her face now. She stated that for the first time in six weeks she actually was able to sleep the whole night. At this point she questions reusing the Kwell treatment."

Reviewed with Dr. S. RESPONSE: "He stated that she needed to wait a full seven days before re-shampooing and using the body lotion of Kwell. He stated that she could use very small amounts on her face but she needed to be careful of eyes, nose, and mouth areas and stay away from those. Pt. today reports a different situation stating that she just has a lot of achy joints, feels that she continues with bites and continues with the itching all over. She did ask to schedule an appointment and to follow-up if this next Kwell treatment didn't cure it and she was placed to scheduling for that appointment."

We put 4,500 labels on the fall sale flyers I picked up. I took the flyers to the bulk mail depot at the post office and then met my birthday group for lunch. It felt strange listening to all the fun chatter with so much facial and head activity going on, but I never let on. How could I possibly explain this?

"Remember that I have commanded you to be determined and confident! Do not be afraid or discouraged, For I, the Lord your God are with you wherever you go." Josh. 1:9 Good News Bible

In my mind I limit you so often Lord. I lose sight of the fact that you are always with me and have given me the gift of your love. Thank you Lord.

I now feel the gathering of enough strength to put one foot in front of the other and continue on in my quest to find a cure. I felt I owed it to Bob, our children, and our parents, who needed me as they moved into old age. If this continued, I would be no help to any of them.

On September 9th, I had an office visit with dermatologist Dr. S. He wrote: "This is a fifty-five-year-old lady who is seen in follow up of fleeting paresthesias of undetermined etiology, which she feels is due to some sort of an ectoparasite. She describes seeing tiny little spots in bath water and on her clothing, etc. I last treated her for scabies. She states that the night she put the lotion on and the next night she slept without any problem and then everything came back. She did in fact have a second treatment. I discussed with her that this would be an uncharacteristic response for scabies and that her description of the symptoms no longer seems to fit that entity at all, and that I had no options for her other than to try to just act as normal as she can. She has apparently been bathing extra times. I think she is probably drying her skin and irritating it. I don't see any evidence for any organic pathology. I just told her to take Periactin at bedtime and see how she did and come back on a PRN basis."

Obviously, my dermatologist was stumped. If I wasn't so sure I was lucid and normal other than my ludicrous physical symptoms, I would have joined in thinking "this lady is off her rocker." But, because I felt a diagnosis and cure had to be just around the corner with the next doctor I saw, I didn't get aggressive with stepping outside the box. I just kept living with the symptoms and hoping that very soon something would show up that would solve this mystery. The problem, I would discover, was that by waiting I was allowing my condition to become systemic.

After my visit with dermatologist Dr. S., I went back to work. Our anniversary sale was going full tilt. I had ordered Gus and Goldie costumes (our company mascots) for two of our employees to wear.

They attracted much attention sitting outside the front of our store waving at cars passing on the highway. Strange to see people-sized fish!

We had a big sales seminar one afternoon with great customer turn out for coffee and cookies, which I set up. Our sales representative was on hand for a pool chemical presentation. My physical symptoms raged while I pretended to be calm and cool, acting like the business professional I had always been before. It was knowing that my late nights were the worst part of my life and knowing what I would face when I got home and went to bed. I dreaded it.

"There is only one limit to what prayer can do- that is what God can do."
R.A. Torrey

"Is anything too hard for the Lord?"
Genesis 18:14 Good News Bible

Why was I so worried? So many things were out of my control now, but I could still pray. And pray I did on my knees saying the rosary, the beautiful prayer Mary the Mother of God gave to us. As Pope Paul VI said, "This simple and profound prayer, the Rosary, teaches us to make Christ the principle and the end, not only of Marian devotion, but of our entire spiritual life."

Mary's rosary is scripturally Christ-centered. I tried to attend morning Mass as often as I could. I mostly just sat there and absorbed the graces flowing. I had a hard time concentrating. Somehow I felt somewhat normal if I could be there at Mass looking normal.

On September 16th I called into the doctor's office.

NURSE NOTES. REASON: "Pt. Called requesting a refill of Kwell. She stated that she did find more relief with the second Kwell treatment and she would like to try it again."

RESPONSE: "This request has been denied but he did approve of the Periactin 4 mg every six hours prn count of twenty called to Walmart Pharmacy."

Perhaps I was grasping at straws, but I did feel the Kwell helped some. At this point it was my only hope. Things really didn't change a lot with the Kwell or the Periactin. I still kept thinking external treatment might help, but, looking back, all of this was a total waste of time. The gremlins were advancing, and the Kwell and Periactin didn't even slow them down.

Shortly after our big fall sale's pitch, I found myself dealing with our estimated taxes due, and I made sure they got in the mail. Our office manager had been on maternity leave, and I didn't feel I wanted to leave this job to her on her first day back. Was it ever nice to have her back, though, as I had been doing many of her duties on top of my own.

"Humble yourselves, then, under God's mighty hand, So that he will lift you up in His own good time. Leave all your worries with him, because He cares for you." I Peter 5:6-7 Good News Bible

This is incredible, Lord and so comforting! Teach me to keep my eyes on you and to allow you to give me peace of heart and mind today. These words were definitely speaking to me today. Thank you, Jesus.

On September 26th, I had another visit with the dermatologist, Dr. S. He wrote: "This is a fifty-five-year-old female who is seen again for complaints of itching and a sensation of a bug biting her and concerned over having ectoparasites. She comes in today stating that she has two spots that she did not have last night when she went to bed.

"Examination shows two small, 1 mm, dark lesions which was just wiped off with a four-by-four and seemed to be dried blood. The other was removed with kind of a skin scraping and under the microscope is, in fact, just a small drop of dry blood. No ectoparasites were seen. She states that she is hoping to get the Kwell again today because they just redid the dogs and they are getting their house fumigated and wants to do this all at once. This would be her third treatment. I did authorize 4 oz. of Kwell Lotion and told her that that would be the last time and if she has further problems that I really could not be of any assistance to her."

Oh, this was just great! I was out in the cold with this doctor and wondering what to do next. I was saddened first to be in this situation but mostly because it was starting to look fairly hopeless. I had obviously done a very poor job of describing my situation as rereading these notes makes it seem so minimal. I was actually totally miserable, scared and very uncomfortable.

After work Bob and I attended our old high-school awards banquet. It was a beautiful evening with dinner, student entertainment, and socializing with friends. Until I had to go home and face the night. And the night was as bad as any other I had recently endured. Very little sleep with raging zips and zags and drilling pain mostly in the back of my head and my torso . . . lots of activity around my eyes and face. Intestinal problems remain. I also continued to observe little black spots on my torso . . . they had what looked like string emerging from them. They could be brushed off but the spot looked bloody.

"For the Spirit that God has given us does not make us timid; instead His Spirit fills us with power, love and discipline."   2 Timothy 1:7 Good News Bible

Lord, whatever I fear most, I give to you; trusting that you will give me your peace and courage.

My doctors told me I was not contagious, but I had worried a lot about this. I decided to trust that God wanted me to continue my life of living and loving, and I would do so whenever and until I was told not to. Obviously I used sterile techniques around people and family and washed my hands and used sanitizers numerous times a day as a precaution.

Chapter Four

Delving Deeper

O N OCTOBER 3RD, 1996, I REQUESTED to see a new doctor who I had great respect for, Internal Medicine Specialist Dr. F.E. Bob and I knew him and his wife socially and also through our business. I prayed that he could somehow figure out what was wrong with me.

I had a 7:30 a.m. breakfast meeting before a busy day at work started. Also I had a doctor's appointment with a doctor I felt would surely see the symptoms I had and know what to do next. I was terribly hopeful.

My appointment was a little strained as I had to present my ridiculous symptoms to a doctor I knew socially and through business. He listened intently but didn't react one way or the other. I felt exhausted.

He wrote, "Conversation with the patient regarding what she terms a parasitic infection. She is going to the University of Minnesota on November 12th. I am going to obtain a CBC and stools for ova and parasites. I will be looking for eosinophilia."

That was it. The short of it. One more hope turned into a very small sentence.

I continued to pray for God's direction.

Our spa sales representative representing Hot Spring Portable Spas from Carlsbad, California, came to visit. Bob and I always enjoyed his visits. He always brought a wealth of data, tested sales techniques, and suggestions. He was pleased with our spa sales.

Even though my body was experiencing drastic changes, I did not have to allow my faith to falter. *Help me Lord*, I prayed continuously.

I made a call to DR. F.E.'s nurse with a question. Since I felt somewhat better when on an antibiotic and I had been researching the role antibiotics played in diseases with similar symptoms as mine, I wanted to ask Dr.F.E. if Trimethoprim could possibly be prescribed. Several of the medical books I perused had listed it as a good antibiotic to use for bacterial infections. Up to this point, neither I nor my doctors had reason to believe I had a bacterial infection, but I was anxious to try this medicine to see if it would bring me relief. I simply needed to function at this point as I had been very ill since July.

NURSE NOTES. REASON: "Patient states she has been doing research at St. Ben's Library. Was wondering if doctor would start her on Trimethoprim. (Note: Trimethoprim is an antibiotic used to treat bacterial infections. I requested it because I always felt better on an antibiotic if only on a temporary basis)"

REVIEWED WITH: Dr. F.E. RESPONSE: "He said she should wait until she goes to the U of M next month. Patient advised."

On October 14, I saw Dr. F.E. again. He wrote in his notes, "Copies of patient's most recent labs, office visits, progress notes, etc are made available for patient pickup this afternoon. See Authorization. Of note, the CBC and stools for ova and parasites were negative."

These records were for the perusal of the University of Minnesota doctors for the appointment I had coming up. I saw some value in taking my records with me, but I didn't think I'd recommend it to others. The records may lead the examiner, and I had no way of knowing if this is what happened.

"Be joyful always, pray at all times, and be thankful in all circumstances. This is what God wants from you in your life in union with Christ Jesus."
I Thes. 5: 16-18 Good News Bible

My morning prayer . . . I really had to think about this one . . . at this point I was having trouble with the "give thanks in all circumstances" part. But when I put things in perspective I still had many things to be thankful for—a loving husband and loving family. Our daughter and son-in-law and son and daughter–in–law are expecting our first grandchildren (in February and April), our business was doing well, all four of our parents were alive and doing well. We also enjoyed the company of many friends and had a fun social life. The list could go on and on.

At the top of my list always was the role God played in my life. I never believed the road to salvation would be easy or expected it to be. This strange illness was a bump in the road to be sure. But bumps don't turn into mountains unless one let them. I was determined to keep my "bump" small enough so I could still see over it.

I had a very busy day at work as our office manager was attending a sales seminar, so I had to do double duty.

I took my blood pressure and it was high for me at 146/100. My usual used to be 100/80.

I was scheduled to see a new doctor at my clinic, another internal medicine specialist, Dr. M. He was very kind and soft-spoken. I could tell he badly wanted to help me but felt as frustrated as I did with the impossible emerging of totally radical symptoms. I had stopped talking about "bugs" as I knew this wouldn't get me anywhere. However, the creepy, crawly, biting continued in force and only abated temporarily when I began a new antibiotic or other prescription medication.

Dr. M. wrote in his notes, "The patient is a fifty-five-year-old woman, who is here to see me for multiple symptoms. She has achiness, fatigue, diffuse itching, occasional needle-like pains, chills, global headaches, frequent loose stools, lack of appetite, fleeting skin rashes, and other symptoms. She states that she has not felt well since July. She blames the initiation of her symptoms on bringing her dog home from an operation at the veterinarian's at the University of Minnesota. She has seen Dr. S several times, as well as Dr. L., for evaluation of 'ectoparasite.'

She received several treatments with Kwell. She had also taken some of her daughter's Bactrim and recently completed a two-week course, 'completely resolved her symptoms.' They returned even worse after discontinuation. She states that currently, her symptoms are predominantly neck aching, headache, and fatigue. There is no more rash. She states that she had seen an eye doctor recently for a 'black discharge from her eyes.' She brought in Q-tips that show remnants of this discharge. She has an appointment scheduled with infectious disease at the University of Minnesota on November 12th, 1996. She normally takes no medications. She is not allergic to any known medications. She and her husband own their own swimming pool and spa distributorship here in St. Cloud. They have not recently traveled out of the country. They have two dogs at home. She has been quite healthy most of her life, except for a broken leg and an evaluation for some transient diarrhea and rectal bleeding. She had a colonoscopy in 1994, which showed only internal hemorrhoids. These symptoms resolved."

PHYSICAL EXAMINATION: "She appears to be a tense, but otherwise pleasant woman, who is in no acute distress. Her blood pressure is 146/100. Her heart rate is normal. Her eyes appear normal. There is no facial rash. There is a vague erythematous rash below her anterior neck bilaterally. This does not blanch. The neck is supple. The chest is clear to auscultation. The heart exam is without murmurs. The abdominal exam reveals no masses, tenderness, or distention. There is no lymphadenopathy palpable in the anterior cervical or posterior cervical areas, or in the axillary or inguinal areas. Her skin is without rash, other than the aforementioned rash on her neck. The neurologic examination, including cranial nerves, strength, and sensation, is normal. There is no diminution of the pulses in her extremities."

LABORATORY STUDIES: "She has had a normal CBC on 10/03/96 and 08/14/96. Stools were negative for O&P on 10/08/96."

ASSESSMENT AND PLAN: "Multisystem illness. With the multiple symptoms, I think some attention needs to be given to checking for systemic diseases. However, these symptoms point me in no specific direction. The patient seems to be quite concerned about the possibility of infection and states that she was back to normal on Bactrim, but frustratingly had a recurrence of her symptoms off the Bactrim. She also believes that there may be a connection to her dogs.

"I don't have any specific conditions in mind. However, I think consideration needs to be given to possible liver disease, thyroid disease, or possibly celiac sprue, with the diarrhea and transient skin lesions, peripheral neuropathy of some kind with the tingling sensation, and certainly psychiatric disease, such as an anxiety disorder or an obsessive compulsive disorder. We'll start with some screening labs with a CBC with an eosinophil count, urinalysis, liver function tests, thyroid function tests and TSH. VDRL and B-12 might be ordered in the future. She wants to have some lab tests to take with her to the University of Minnesota. I did not broach the idea that we may not be able to find out what is causing her symptoms. I do not feel that empiric antibiotics are warranted. I think this disappointed her. I think this is going to take some time and some testing yet to find out what is going on. It may be that we will not come up with a firm answer, and then we'll have to broach possible psychiatric causes of this syndrome. Certainly, a thorough medical evaluation is warranted at this point, but I am skeptical that we will find an underlying condition."

Dr. E.M. (November 7, 1996) As a correction to these doctor's notes, I will add that Bob and I took a trip to Cancun, Mexico, January 29th to February 2nd, 1996. I also traveled to Houston, Texas, to visit my sister Jayne and family from February 24th to February 28th, 1996, and became very ill there. I lost eight pounds and experienced intestinal distress. No one else I was in contact with got anything, which I was grateful for.

"CERTAINLY PSYCHIATRIC DISEASE, SUCH AS AN ANXIETY DISORDER OR AN OBSESSIVE COMPULSIVE DISORDER." Okay, the cat's out of the bag.

I knew it didn't go well as the look of disbelief permeated Dr. E.M.'s demeanor as I tried to state my case calmly. After I read these doctor notes, I realized it actually was much worse than I surmised. Thank heavens I did not hear the words "psychiatric disease," "anxiety disorder" or "obsessive compulsive disorder." They might have paralyzed me from taking the future actions I ended up taking. I might have started actually questioning myself. When these words are used (and so often they are in these types of cases) the words are sometimes self-fulfilling.

Lunch with my birthday group was next on my agenda for the day. Lunch was good, as it was always fun and comforting to hear all the chatter and small talk and what was on everybody's minds. I loved my good friends but could not bring myself to share my very embarrassing story. Somehow I couldn't help but wonder if any of them could possibly top my dilemma. It was a real doozy.

Back to work. Busy day. Bank deposits, payroll, and taxes to do.

I was also helping my daughter purchase furniture for her home. We didn't talk about my health issues. At this point better that way.

That night was very difficult. Hardly any sleep. But I found comfort in the knowledge that God knew and cared about me and had a plan that I was not yet aware of.

"I am a God who is everywhere and not in one place only. No one can hide where I cannot see him. Do you not know that I am everywhere in Heaven and on earth."   Jer. 23:23-24 Good News Bible

I called Dr. M.'s nurse on November 6th.

NURSE NOTES. REASON: "Patient called this morning stating that she is having exploding loose stools. She had one through the night, one at 6:30 this morning and one at 9:30 this morning. She is wondering if Dr. M would prescribe the same medication that (Gastroenterologist) Dr. H had prescribed to her in the past when she had a diagnosis of colitis, stating that this med worked great and would like to consider using this medication again.

REVIEWED with Internal Medicine Specialist Dr. E.M.

RESPONSE: "He states that he would prefer not to order antibiotic at this time, that meds may interfere with her appointment that she has scheduled at the U of M Hospital and patient is vocalizing concern that she would like to cancel the appointment at the U of M and try antibiotics. I have reviewed this with Dr. M again, and he has spoken to the patient in regard to this and a new prescription has been called to Wal-Mart for E-Mycin 250mg qid, #40, and patient will call after completion of this regimen if she is having further concerns."

Obviously I needed to keep my appointment at the U but being so sick, I was ready to grasp at anything and antibiotics seemed my only hope. They were a temporary fix at best but temporary seemed to be the most I could hope for those days.

November 11, 1996. Because all the doctors told me I was not contagious and none of my family members, friends, or co-workers got sick, I did not avoid contact with other people and continued all normal activities as best I could. I did however use sterile technique as much as possible.

Our whole family celebrated Bob's birthday at our lake cabin over the weekend. I made all the food as I usually do because I love to cook. But I was exhausted and could hardly climb the twelve stairs to the second floor without stopping to rest. Until this past summer I could easily run up them.

Back at work found me busier than usual because I had plans to be off the next day to go to the U of M for an all-day appointment with Dr. S. at the Infectious Disease office. I was so hopeful that a specialist could finally get to the bottom of my condition. Having worked at the university as an registered nurse in the critical care, dermatology, kidney, heart, and cancer floor, I had seen many unusual and difficult cases. Doctors referred their sickest patients to us from a five-state area. I remembered taking care of a man from North Dakota with a severely advanced skin disease. Sadly nothing could ever be found to help him and the doctors and nurses tried everything. I often wondered what happened to him as he was still a patient when I left the floor to have our first child. I thought of him often as I now was battling something that at times mimicked his condition. Horror of all horrors—his body had deteriorated to such an extent that he looked less than human. Was I next?

Due to the multiple problems with my eyes, I made an appointment with Eye Surgeons and Physicians to be evaluated. My first appointment resulted in a prescription for Tobradex.

EYE DOCTOR NOTES: Phone conversation: "Eyes better. Tobradex has helped a lot. But black mattering every morning. Patient asked, 'Would culturing the eye exudate be helpful in making RX for this systemic illness problems going on?' Has an appointment at U of M next week for complete physical. She will let us know if anything comes up that we should know about.

I called Dr. M.'s nurse again on November 11th.

NURSE NOTES. REASON: "Patient called stating that she would like to speak with Dr. E.M., stating that her sister is a nurse practitioner and has further information to share with Dr. E.M. States again also that she is having further loose stools. She was on Erythromycin after two days and those stools reappeared. She will be keeping appointment with U of M physician tomorrow. Copy of labs has been picked up by patient for her to take with her to appointment at U of M Hospital."

Another bad night with determination to keep fighting the next day.

My nurse practitioner sister Sue tried her hardest to make sense of my symptoms and suggested various tests. Throughout these last four months, we have had numerous discussions. She was as perplexed as I was. When I told her the doctors did not seem to believe I had a disease but were alluding to a psychiatric diagnosis she simply said, "But you have symptoms!"

I indeed did, more numerous as each day went by. I was getting physically sicker and sicker with no explainable diagnosis on the horizon. At times I wondered, if this keeps up how I could go on with any semblance of a normal life? That was a dark thought I tried hard to suppress.

"Never confuse the will of the majority with the will of God."
Charles Colson.

"Do not conform yourselves to the standards of this world, but let God transform you inwardly by a complete change of your mind. Then you will be able to know the will of God what is good and is pleasing to Him and is perfect."
Romans 12:2 Good News Bible

I was gradually reaching the conclusion that the medical community might not be able to help me. I might have to think outside the box and not conform to the established patterns of this country. But for now, I was trusting in the expertise of the U of M doctors and was excited to be able to consult with them.

On November 12th, I spent the day at the University of Minnesota (Infectious Disease) with Dr. S. in hopes of getting a diagnosis. Bob accompanied me. Before my appointment, we met our two sons for lunch in Minneapolis. Small talk was the norm, but I could sense a curiosity about why I felt the need to see a doctor at the U. I had not shared a lot of information regarding my symptoms with them. I was worried enough and felt no need to involve my children at this point. So I minimized the reason for my visit and then quietly sat through lunch with symptoms raging and listened to the small talk between Bob and our sons.

Dr. S. spent quite a bit of time with me, and he was very thorough, but I could tell he had no experience with any patient quite like me. He carefully listened to my story and did not seem to be alarmed. He ordered a battery of tests. He asked if stool cultures were ever done in St. Cloud. Yes, they had been, I reported. Numerous times. I had a good work-up and blood work, but there was to be no solution available to me from this visit.

I went home with a twenty-four-hour urine test. I went home fairly dejected. Actually correction—extremely dejected. I was starting to see I may have to step outside the medical community box in order to get well. But as a conventionally trained R.N., I had absolutely no idea on how to go about that process.

After returning from the U, I made notes regarding how I felt: Present were the following—sharp pain in my right ankle . . . ankle on the same leg where I had broken the tibia and fibula years before that had never given me any trouble. I had tightness across my chest, throat clogged up, a dull ache behind my right ear, sharp pains into groin area, a stiff neck, and a headache. What an unusual conglomerate of symptoms.

I called Dr. H.'s office on November 14th.

NURSE NOTES. REASON: "Patient called this morning stating she would like me to check with Dr. H. (A gastroenterologist she had seen previously). Would like prescription for Asacol, which she has taken in the past. (Note: RX for frequent diarrhea) She states she was taking two tablets every four hours, stating this has helped her. Diarrhea is so miserable for her at the present time and through the conversation, she then states she would like prescription for Flagyl (RX for treating infections that are strongly suspected to be caused by bacteria), not the Asacol, and would like me to speak with Dr. H. I have explained to her that I need to speak with Dr. E.M. in regard to this and he will, in turn, decide if Dr.H needs to be consulted. She states that University of Minnesota is doing a general work-up for her at the present time."

RESPONSE: "He desires that she continue her regimen of EES and after those Flagyl 250 mg tid, #30, is to be taken by the patient. I have called this prescription into Wal-Mart per the patient's request and she verbalizes understanding to complete the regimen of the EES. Big concern with her now, she would like stool cultures done to rule out parasites from *Capillaria aerophilia*, stating that she has spoken with someone in microbiology at the U of M and they feel that three stools need to be obtained, skipping one day apart in-between these and to specifically specify that they need to be tested for *Capillaria aerophilia*. This has been reviewed with Dr. E.M. and he states he would like to either speak with patient's veterinarian for her dog or would like a copy of the report from that visit. Patient's veterinarian is Dr. N., and Karen will call Dr. N. and have these records sent to clinic for Dr. E.M.to review. (It does not appear that any of these records were ever sent to Dr. E.M.) I did Call Dr. N, the veterinarian, and requested that she do that.

My request to rule out *Capillaria aerophilia* was because our Bichon Lacey's vet found an adult worm football shaped in her stool. She said it was very rare, and she had never seen one before.

Interestingly, Lacey developed a myriad of symptoms simultaneously. (At the same time that I was struggling with some of the same symptoms.) Also we began our initial symptoms on the same day.

These were some of the symptoms she had: Extreme exudate dark matter from her eyes, extreme weakness, weight loss, diarrhea, itching and scratching, arthritis-type symptoms, vomiting.

At first with all the itching and stinging and biting, I assumed she had fleas. But I never did find a flea. I used many flea removal agents on the market and shampooed her many times. Our home was fumigated, and bed clothes were washed many, many times.

I took Lacey in for many veterinarian visits. Her vet tried various medications.

The fact that we got sick at the same time really seemed like too much of a coincidence. This fact never seemed to interest any of the medical people I saw.

Her veterinarian never did give her a diagnosis either. Because she became totally debilitated, we needed to put her to sleep in 1999.

Tears of great sadness flowed to say goodbye to my beloved dog. Sadness overcame me because I had been powerless to help her and confronted the certainty that I could not even help myself.

I worked all day on November 14th, but I felt so unbelievably tired that I needed to go home to nap several times.

I woke up at 2:00 a.m. with matting, tiny fluttering and pain around my eyes, ears, nose, and throat. I spent most of the night on the couch not to disturb Bob. These physical disturbances did not allow me to sleep. I tossed and turned a great deal plus got up every twenty minutes or so. In the morning, I had a lot of pain in my knee joints, and my neck was stiff and achy. In addition I felt very weak and suffered backache, chills, nausea, and even had difficulty swallowing.

NURSE NOTES on November 15th. REASON: "Karen faxed note to me this morning in regard to her concerns over the parasite that she feels has been transmitted to her by her dog. Please see copy of the fax in the chart. Also, she is calling this morning. She is complaining of joint pain. She is weak and having back pain. She is having loose stools. Is further concerned in regard to treatment for this parasite, stating that she will be picking up literature from her veterinarian regarding the treatment for her dog from the ailment this summer. I have explained to her that Dr. E.M. would like to speak with her veterinarian in regard to this. He will be doing this after he receives the information in regard to treatment for her dogs this morning. Veterinarian is Dr. N. Dr. E.M. will attempt to make contact with the veterinarian. Karen also did drop information off at the clinic this afternoon for Dr. M. to review in regard to the capillariasis. Dr.E. M. has reviewed this information. He states he has reviewed this in the past as well and did read the faxed note from Karen this morning and will attempt to contact the veterinarian."

I never did hear if a conversation took place or if a link was ever considered. I have to assume that my doctor felt there was no connection to the veterinarian's finding. It would have been nice to have some mention made in my doctor notes regarding this.

On November 15th, I woke up at 2:00 a.m. again this night with eyes matting and tiny pains around eyes, ears, nose, and throat. Because I was up and down all night, I spent most of the night on the couch, as usual.

In the morning I noticed lots of pain in knee joints and considerable amount of white string-like discharge in urine. My neck was stiff and aching, I felt general weakness, had a backache, chills, nausea with difficulty swallowing and explosive diarrhea.

I continued on Erythromycin and also Flagyl.

By November 15th, I assessed my situation and knew I needed a plan. I decided to start my plan at our three local libraries: St. John's University, Collegeville, Minnesota; St. Benedict's, St. Joseph, Minnesota; and the St. Cloud Public Library.

Starting at the St. Benedict's library, I parked my car about eighty feet from the main entrance. Now I was walking with great difficulty as my joint pain and lethargy had become pronounced. It was all I could do to walk from my car to the St. Ben's Library. I felt so foggy. When I entered the complex, I asked for directions to the "Medical Reference" area. Stacking up six to eight books on a desk, I got out my legal notebook. I had a long list of my current symptoms and used it to cross-reference anything that sounded like a condition. Many of my symptoms were present all of the time, and others came and went. I never seemed to know when which would happen.

1. Sharp pain in ankle joint (site of a former break of my tibia and fibula) that never bothered me before.
2. Tightness across the chest.
3. Throat feels clogged up.
4. Ache behind ear . . . uncontrolled bleeding several times near ear. It took me ten minutes to stop the bleeding during one bleed.
5. Sharp pains in groin area.
6. Stiff neck-aching (got worse right after I began any of my treatment programs and then better for a while).
7. Headache.
8. Considerable black filamentous matter stuck onto whites of eyes especially in morning. I could feel it moving in my eye at times. Eyes twitch and itch and are bloodshot. I have a harder time focusing. Developed dry eye and cysts on my conjunctiva.
9. Sharp bites (twinges) and then tiny bloody red spots on my skin at site of bite.
10. Tiny bite sensations on face, sensation of crawling around eyes, ears, nose and throat. Wakes me up.
11. Severe pain in knee joints.
12. White string like discharge in urine.
13. Weakness in arms, wrists and legs.

14. Back ache all over; feels like a bad case of the flu.
15. Chills alternate with feverish symptoms.
16. Nausea.
17. Difficulty swallowing.
18. Heart racing. Blood pressure up. Normal used to be 100/80 now up to 160/90.
19. Throat coated with whitish discharge. White, slimy, stringy matter in mouth and nose, almost two inches in length observed at night. Wakes me up. I gargle and it sticks to my tongue. (I used a combination of hydrogen peroxide, saline and aloe to remove it so I could get back to sleep.)
20. Weight loss.
21. Fine tremor of hands (at times I could hardly hold a piece of paper).
22. Easy fatigue.
23. Hair falling out in big clumps and very dry and brittle.
24. Muscular fatigue.
25. Changes in bowel habits: diarrhea, sometimes explosive, and white kernels present in stool.
26. Large red sores on torso and abdomen.
27. Blotchy skin—reddened- —rash like.
28. Irritability.
29. Sadness.
30. Nervousness.
31. Severe Insomnia—so tired and up three to four times a night. Sleep four to five hours a night at most, usually on the couch.
32. Pain across chest, mostly into right area but also left.
33. Arthritis-type pain in right shoulder, legs, knees, and hips.
34. Ear aches.
35. Weakness. I can hardly walk up stairs.
36. Sore eyes—aching, blood shot, yellowish tinge to white area.
37. Severe itching all over.
38. Drilling pain in back of head especially at night when lying down.
39. Black, blue and yellowish spots on body especially legs.

40. Black fibers discovered after a severe itch on torso.
41. Three to six months after onset—swelling in ankles.
42. Three to six months after onset—inability to hold urine when bladder full. No control.
43. Eyes itch in intervals throughout the day, sometimes feeling like squiggles, like something is actually moving. Dark mucous-like matter still forms often, and it sometimes clings to white of eyes. Need to wipe out fifteen to twenty-five times a day.
44. Big toe toenails first developed rough ridges and lines across the nails and then both toenails fell off.

After a few hours at the St. Ben's Library, I realized I needed to focus on the infectious disease area. I scrutinized the *Oxford Companion to Medicine/Intestinal Diseases* Parasitic Ref. R. 12108819686. A section by Dr. K. caught my eye. He had worked in third-world countries and had experience with parasitic infections in humans. The symptoms he listed so closely matched mine I was astonished. It was noted he now had a practice in Canada. (I found the number and called him.) His receptionist answered, and I explained how I came across Dr. K. from an article he wrote in the *Oxford Companion*. She put me through to him, and he graciously answered the phone and listened to my many questions about human parasitic infection.

Could my symptoms have any relation to—
1. *Capillaria aerophilla* (a rare football-shaped egg our vet found in our dog Lacey's stool).
2. Any relationship to a small black insect?
3. What are the methods of transmittal?
4. Possible insect bite?
5. Any relationship to a nematode of some kind?
6. What are the typical symptoms in humans? Dogs? Cats? Others?
7. Have you heard of eye, ear, nose, and throat involvement with dark matter coming out of the eyes?

8. Can parasitic infections be fatal?

9. Is it possible to have an organism move out of the body through the skin? I sometimes noticed a sharp bite then a tiny red spot (bloody) on my skin, then tiny black flying insects would appear. Any connection at all or just a co-incidence?

10. What relationship if any to Trypanosomes, a parasite in the blood and spinal fluid of man and other vertebrates? A Trypanosome is a microscopic one-celled animal. One kind causes African sleeping sickness; others cause other diseases. A Trypanosome is long and thin with a whip-like extension at one end called a flagellum. It also has a thin waving membrane down the length of its body. Many Trypanosomes spend part of their lives inside certain insects.

This multitude of questions seemingly unrelated must have taken him aback. He declined to give me specific medical answers and advice over the telephone, but he did say, "If you were my patient, I would put you on Albendazole."

I knew this was a safe anti-parasitic medication. I thanked him for his time and thought about how I would present this to my new internist.

What I should have done was book a flight to Canada and see this doctor in person. The brain fog never allowed me to think of such a simple solution. And negotiating the Canadian Health System seemed a formidable task.

I called my new internist, Dr. M., and told him about my conversation with Dr. K. (the author of the *Oxford Companion* article) and his suggestion of Albendazole as a prescription. He hesitated and said, no, there simply was no proof of a parasitic infection.

"Faith came singing into my room and other guests took flight. Grief, anxiety, fear and gloom, speed out into the night."   Elizabeth Cheney

Lord, this day may I stay close to you and rest in the calmness of your presence.

"Leave your troubles with the Lord, and he will defend you; he never lets honest men be defeated."   PS 55:22 Good News Bible

Sometimes all I can pray is a simple "Help me, Jesus." My prayers are getting shorter now and more pleading. Looking back, I feel He was quietly holding me up. I do know I received strength that I never knew I had.

On November 16th, I drove sixty miles to our second store to take over because the manager had asked for the day off. It was a busy day with customers. Very hard to keep a smile on my face. I closed up the store and drove home contemplating my situation while the stinging, stabbing and drilling sensations moved around my body.

Sleepless night again . . . up at 3:00 a.m., 4:30 a.m. and 6:00 a.m. and awake lots in between. I was having considerably more trouble with sensations of crawling, tiny bite sensations on my face, eyes, ears, and nose, difficulty swallowing, and a neck ache.

I must keep my focus on the cross and the immense agony Jesus faced to save me and all of His children. My little discomfort was nothing compared to that. I hoped by writing these words my children and grandchildren and all other readers would know this truth in their hearts as well.

On November 17th, we went to the cabin with some of our family to spend the weekend. I cooked, cleaned and tried to act normal so as not to worry them, but I was not well and was anxious to hear of any results from my consultation with Dermatology Dr. S. from the University of Minnesota. Dr. S. called me there, and I held my breath with anticipation of hearing anything at all that could be construed as a diagnosis. As before, when I started on antibiotics, and this time added Flagyl, I felt better, so I told him this. I said I was ninety-percent better, had less eye discharge but still felt weak, especially in my arms, wrists, and legs, and still had an aching neck. I could hardly climb up the stairs at the lake even though before all this I usually took the stairs at a run with no trouble. Dr. S. asked if stool cultures had ever been done in St. Cloud. I said yes. He then informed me that he found my thyroid hormone to be abnormally high. I felt almost glad that something had been found, but I knew that a high thyroid reading probably wouldn't cause all of my strange symptoms. But finally we could treat something. He said he would return the call when the twenty-four-hour urine and other tests came back.

That night was usual with being awake from 3:00 to 3:45 and then 4:30 to 5:00 and then 6:00 to 6:30 and lots in between. I had multiple tiny crawling, bite sensations on face, eyes, ears and nose, difficulty swallowing, and a very sore neck.

The next night, I was up again four times with the same symptoms but in addition, my heart was racing, I felt a lump in my throat, and my throat was coated with whitish matter.

"To have Faith is to be sure of the things we hope for, to be certain of the things we cannot see."   Heb. 11:1 Good News Bible

I wondered how people without faith handled an impossible illness. God helped me focus on the hope and certainty He gave me for eternal salvation. My path here had been a way towards Him. I didn't need always to be content here, and sometimes I could be downright miserable.

Chapter Five

Questions and
More Questions

O N NOVEMBER 18, 1996, I CALLED Dr. E.M. again and asked
if he would reconsider prescribing Albendazol (recommenda-
tion of Dr. K. infectious disease doctor in the Oxford Companion). I also requested more cultures of eyes, ears, nose, throat, and
tongue. I asked if I had been checked for Lymes or Rickettsial infections.

To the nurses and doctors treating me, I know I had to look like a
hypochondriac. I was all over the map with crazy symptoms and even cra-
zier suggestions.

I was very busy at work. I gathered sales totals to prepare the
sales tax due in two days. Lots of catch-up work to do. I continued to
need to go home for naps. I was unbelievably tired all the time. I also
continued to spend quite a bit of time on research.

I called the Parasitology Lab at the University of Minnesota and
asked the tech if they could look outside the box for unusual diseases.
Specifically, might they find ova, helminths, or cryptosporidium in any
samples I sent? I also asked if they knew of any diseases that passed from
animals to people. No definitive answer.

I called an epidemiologist, John Clare, at the Minnesota Public
Health Department to ask if anything unusual was recently reported in
the way of infectious diseases. Answer: No.

I called the Minnesota Department of Health and talked to a veterinarian, J.C., regarding any report of unusual diseases being reported?
His answer like so many others was no. My frustrations levels were ris-
ing.

I called the Mayo Clinic and talked to a nurse in the Infectious Disease department. I reviewed my symptoms with her, and she asked if I'd had bacterial cultures done and had my sputum checked for eggs? I would have to check.

I wondered if I should go to the Mayo Clinic for another workup but decided against it for the time being. It appeared I had something not in medical text books. I was concerned that I may get caught in the delusional trap with them as well.

I honestly didn't know what else to do other than just accept my situation and wait until I got sicker and sicker when my diagnosis, I hoped, might become obvious. I was not so much afraid for myself but did worry about possibly not being here for Bob, my children, future grandchildren, and of course our four elderly parents.

I decided to keep fighting.

"I am the God of your Father Abraham. Do not be afraid; I am with you."
Genesis 26:24 Good News Bible

NURSE NOTES: REASON: "Patient called this morning stating she has been taking Flagyl for approximately two days, and her loose stools continue. She also has not completed her series of the Erythromycin (but will resume it) after talking with a pharmacist about whether she can take both at the same time. She is also asking for another antibiotic at the present time . . . (Actually Albendazole)"

RESPONSE: "Office visit has been scheduled for tomorrow, November 19th for Internal Medicine Specialist Dr. E.M. to speak to patient in further depth."

I next called to make an appointment with my OB doctor, Dr. F. He had been my only doctor for so many years. I felt he knew my history of being a non-complaining person and would listen to my multiple symptoms and be able to refer me to a medical expert or clinic. He could see me on November 21.

I called Dr. E.M. and asked whether I had been checked for Lymes? He said I had hypothyroidism and would need to be treated. I already knew that as the Infectious Disease doctor from the University of Minnesota had given me my thyroid results.

Google Search states that hypothyroidism is a condition when there is a deficiency of thyroid hormone in the body. Hyperthyroidism is characterized by excessive amounts of thyroid hormone in the body. Both hypothyroidism and hyperthyroidism are extremely different cases. The signs and symptoms of hyperthyroidism include increased activity of bowel movements, difficulty in sleeping, intolerance to heat, nervousness and palpitation, increased respiratory rate, increased moisture of the skin, increased metabolic rate, soft and fine hair, wandering mind, sweating, scanty menstrual periods, infertility, muscle weakness, nervousness, and soft nails.

In hypothyroidism there are symptoms such as bradycardia, decreased heart rate, constipation, intolerance to cold, memory problems, coarse dry hair, slow speech, slow walking movements, dry skin, brittle nails, weight gain, fatigue, irritability, infertility, puffy face, loss of eyebrow hair, and heavy menstrual periods.

My symptoms were not entirely characteristic of either of these thyroid conditions, but I trusted the test results so was willing to be treated for hypothyroidism.

I again asked the doctor if he would consider prescribing Albendazol (anti-parasitic) as mentioned by the *Oxford Companion* doctor, but he ignored my request. Oh, well, at least I would be treated for something.

I prepared a summary of the onset of my disease to explain to my obstetrician Dr. F. in a couple of days.

On November 19th, I had my office visit wth Dr. E.M., an internal medicine specialist. He wrote: "The patient is here for follow-up today. We are working together to try and solve what sounds like a multi-system illness. Her symptoms are currently predominated by fatigue, malaise, and frequent loose stools. She has not had any fevers. She has had no skin changes. She has noticed a dark exudate that she wipes out of her eyes each morning. She also describes transient prickling or biting pains that occur mostly in her shoulders and above.

"The patient has been mostly focused on an infection. She has been talking with a parasitologist in Canada and has also been seen by an infectious disease consultant in the Twin Cities. She believes that she has been infected by something and that if she is without antibiotics, then she does poorly. After our last meeting, I agreed to treat her with an empiric course of antibiotics for the possibility of bacterial overgrowth of her small bowel. We started with Erythromycin for ten days and she is now on three days of Flagyl. She states when she stops taking the medication, she immediately feels worse. She says, 'I have to take the antibiotics to be able to work.'

"There is no history of thyroid disease. She denies any cold intolerance. Her last menses were three years ago. A TSH was done on her last visit and was 7.36. I had not seen this result, as it somehow had not come past my desk or to my nurse's desk. Apparently, they got a similar result in the Twin Cities."

After my physical with him, Dr. E.M. wrote: "On exam today, she is nervous and tearful at times. Her weight is 122 pounds, which is stable. Her blood pressure is 140/78. There is no tremor. Her eyes appear normal. On close inspection, there is no conjunctivitis and no exudate from the lacrimal ducts. Her oral pharynx is normal. The TM's are normal. There is no thyromegaly. On careful inspection, there are no nodules. There is no cervical lymphadenopathy. The chest is clear to auscultation. There are no heart murmurs. The abdominal examination is also normal. There is no pedal edema. Her EKG today shows a normal sinus rhythm with a regular rate. She does have some T-wave abnormalities in the inferior and anterolateral leads. These were present in 1986. Stool cultures were ordered and are pending."

In his assessment and plan, he wrote: "Multi-system illness. I firmly believe many of her symptoms can be explained by hypothyroidism. I apologized for not getting the information to her sooner that she was hypothyroid. I really discouraged her from focusing on parasitic or another infectious disease. She does request a Lyme titer, and I will do this today. I will also follow up with liver tests to check if there has been any change. We started a dose of Synthroid. I advised her that she may feel much better over the next few weeks. She persistently requested Albendazole for a possible parasitic infection, specifically *Caprillaria aerophila*. I told her that I would have to have at least some suggestion that she had a parasitic infection even to prescribe a safe medicine like Albendazole. I will meet with her again in three weeks.

"I also spoke with her daughter this morning, who voiced concerns about her mother. The daughter states that her mother is not the type to seek out medical help unless she absolutely needs it. I told the daughter that I would continue working with her mother and do what tests I felt were appropriate."

I very much appreciated my daughter going to bat for me. I needed my doctor to see that someone who knew me well believed I was not delusional. My daughter is a registered nurse completing her degree at the College of St. Catherine in 1996.

I wish I could share Dr. M.'s enthusiasm for the end benefits of treating the hypothyroidism with Synthroid. I still maintain that the hypothyroidism is a *result* of my infectious disease and the most alarming symptoms cannot be cured with Synthroid. Only time will tell.

The nurse also wrote up notes. "Patient was in to see Dr. E.M. Prescriptions have been called into Wal-Mart per his request. They were written and are called in for Synthroid for hypothyroidism, with three additional refills and Restoril for insomnia, with no additional refills."

Okay, these medical people thought nothing much was wrong with me. I was just supposed to get over it. I only wish it were that easy to do.

"Most folks are about as happy as they make up their minds to be."
Abraham Lincoln

I love this thought by President Lincoln. I would try to be as happy as I could while fighting for a cause and cure. Maybe all this happened for a reason; someday I might be able to help others in the same or similar predicament.

On November 19th, Dr. E.M. ordered more blood work, including Lymes titer and prescribed Synthroid and Temazepam for my sleep issues. I stayed on the Terazepam for only a couple of weeks as it didn't make any difference. He also ordered Hemoccult II Sensa stool test for blood in stool due to diarrhea since July and took a chest x-ray and EKG. All these tests, sadly, were negative. What do I do now?

On November 21st, I had a busy morning at work. I was looking forward to seeing my OB-Gyn doctor to whom I had gone for over twenty years. I figured he knew me so well, he would not categorize my symptoms as possibly related to a psychosis. After all, my chart was so thin. I never had many complaints and saw him once a year for my usual Pap and checkup. I was sure, even though he was an OB-Gyn, he would know who to send me to for a diagnosis and then treatment.

My appointment was a disaster. I laboriously recanted my last four months of struggle with this unknown thing. He listened quietly. I watched him, determined to not react but forming a clear impression. There would be no small talk during this visit. After I finished, he calmly, said, "Have you considered taking the Minnesota Multiphasic?"

I knew this test was used by trained professionals to assist in identifying personality structure and psychopathology. A huge lump formed in my throat as his words seeped into my understanding. This was a test to rule out mental illness. He didn't believe what I was telling him.

Could I be hearing correctly? How could he possibly jump to this conclusion after our twenty-year history? I had no idea modern medical schools had such a narrow frame of reference to diagnosing diseases, especially those with actual physical symptoms. Didn't he remember how normal I'd always been?

As a nurse I knew what he meant and could hardly believe my ears . . . he actually thought I needed to be evaluated for a psychiatric condition!

I would have expected this from any other doctor, but I was shocked by this attitude because Dr. F. knew me so well. I rarely called him between yearly visits, and complaints were few. How could he not see my systemic symptoms?

These four months of being brave came to a screeching halt right there in the doctor's office, and I burst into tears. Yes, I know, some might say this was an a-typical menopausal woman's response. He looked kindly at me, and all I could say, tight-lipped, was "I'll look into it."

Our visit was over, and so was our twenty-year relationship. I stopped at the desk on my way out and asked his receptionist, my long-time friend Alice, for my records, as I was no longer coming back. I could not possibly waste my time—nor his—in the future. I had major work to do and could not be distracted by psychiatric testing or the impenetrable wall of disbelief. I would continue to search for a diagnosis with my internist, but I had very little hope there as well.

"As long as the world exists, there will be a time for planting, and a time for harvest. There will always be cold and heat, summer and winter, day and night."   Genesis 8:22 Good News Bible

There also will be joy and pain, and I am squarely in the middle of a pain part . . . how far away is the joy? Help me dear Jesus.

When it became clear to me that the medical community was absolutely unable to get to the bottom of my strange illness, I knew I needed to go it alone. I hoped and prayed I would have the strength to do the research, the coherence to interpret the results, and then the ability to find the cure. I also felt in my weakened condition I might be a candidate for a serious illness to strike that would have a diagnosis. I was quite weak by that point with major symptoms and trying to hold up my end of the business and our family and friends and Bob. It took super-human effort to keep a smile on my face and continue to say, "I'm just fine," when a customer or friend asked "How are you?" I knew instinctively that if I allowed my demeanor to crack, all would be lost. I had to stay strong and focused. I had a big job ahead of me. I was also on my knees in prayer throughout the day and night.

Chapter Six

Multiple Symptoms—
Still No Diagnosis

On November 22nd, 1996, I had an appointment with Dr. H., of Eye Surgeons and Physicians. Dr. H. was a family friend. I so appreciated his trying to help me pin this strange disease down, at least related to the eye involvement, plus multiple other physical anomalies.

He wrote, "Still mattering [my eyes], redness gone . . . on to-bradex ointment and natural tears. Patient wants culture. To lab for eye cultures and stool cultures."

On the 27th, I had a follow-up. Dr. M., a colleague of Dr. H. wrote, "Ova and parasites on ears and eyes ordered by Dr. H—'look for capillaria.' No ova and parasites seen. No bacteria seen. Culture: Staphylococcus, coagulase negative, grown on subculture. Mic/sensitivity not done. No fungus grown after nine days. Specimens examined were eye, nasal secretion and saliva."

That day I also had an office visit with Internal Medicine Dr. E.M. He wrote, "Karen is here for a follow-up visit. This is a fifty-four-year-old lady with multiple symptoms that we have been trying to put together. We had diagnosed her with hypothyroidism and have started Synthroid replacement. She is feeling somewhat better with less tremulousness, less weakness, and less diffuse pain. She still, however, feels like she has the flu and feels like she may be getting bronchitis. She is currently only taking Synthroid. She is still very concerned that she has a parasite that she picked up from her dog. She has seen an eye doctor, Dr. H., and he is ordering a culture of the exudate from her eyes and had actually ordered stool cultures to be done. I had ordered that to be done in our clinic but apparently the patient received hem-occults. She has delivered two stools to the lab. However, they have been sitting in her car for long periods and are probably not fresh enough to be analyzed."

After his physical examination, he wrote, "Her vital signs are normal. She appears well but is almost tearful at times. Her oropharynx is normal. The neck is normal. Chest is clear. Heart examination is normal. Abdominal examination is without masses. Skin is without abnormalities. No labs are done today."

I was not surprised at his assessment. "Multiple symptoms. I emphasized the need to try to obtain a diagnosis first. There is really no evidence at this point for a parasitic infection. In fact, her eosinophil's have been normal as have most of her labs. She is quite afraid to travel without antibiotics, and I agreed to supply her with some Keflex to be taken in case of bronchitis symptoms. This seems to be the only way she will feel comfortable going on a bus trip to Branson, Missouri. We will see what her stool cultures show. I don't think the exudate from her eyes is going to be anything that leads to a pathological diagnosis.

Then came the nurse's notes. "Patient was notified that lab tests from November 19 were within normal limits. The absolute eos, Lyme disease, total protein, albumin, T4, SGOT, direct bilirubin, CPX, WBC, and hemoglobin as well as chest x-ray all were within normal limits. Patient states she is feeling some better. She is not having as much pain in her chest and her arms, stating the weakness in her legs has decreased. She is having some problems with insomnia; she is up three to four times to the bathroom in regard to the loose stools. She is stating she is seeing her eye doctor, Dr. H., in regard to the dark circles around her eyes. She is collecting samples from her eyes as well as collecting stool samples. She states she has been working with the lab in regard to these. Also, patient is leaving for a bus tour to Branson, Missouri, on Friday, November 29th along with her husband and friends. She is asking if Dr. M. would order a broad spectrum antibiotic for this just as a prophylactic in case she needs it, stating that she at times will get a stiff neck and become weak. She states she has been on Amoxicillin, Flagyl, and Erythromycin in the past."

The doctor response was, "He states that prior to ordering antibiotic, he would desire to see patient in the office. An appointment has been scheduled this afternoon for 4:45 p.m.

Overall I enjoyed the trip to Branson, but I experienced multi-symptoms continuously throughout. I slept almost continuously while on the bus, but then the nights were a nightmare. It's hard to be quiet in a motel room when so many symptoms are raging and Bob was trying to sleep. In between I tried to be normal. I had actually gotten pretty good at it. A new symptom was my hugely edematous legs. Now what was that about? Maybe that was caused by the long intervals of riding the bus.

"Come ye thankful people, come, raise the song of harvest home; God our maker doth provide for our wants to be supplied; come to God's own temple, come, raise the song of harvest home."
Henry Alford

I reminded myself to be thankful even for today. If I had to be so sick somewhere I might as well be on a scenic bus tour to Branson!

On December 5th, I called in to the office of the internal medicine specialist, Dr. E.M. The nurse's notes read, "The patient called stating she would like lab results from last office visit. Stated that while she was on her trip, she needed to start antibiotics as she was ill. Concerned about her blood pressure. Normal blood pressure for her is 110/80. She had checked it while on her trip and it was 149/104. She stated also that she received the results of the eye cultures from eye doctor Dr. H. and that they were negative. She is complaining of her ankles being very edematous, but they were really, really bad while she was on her trip. They are somewhat better today. Also concerned that her hands and arms are tingling. She also states she has dark mucous drainage from her eyes. Questioned whether serology studies have been done at this point, stating that she has spoken with a friend who is in a lab, and she is suggesting that serology testing be done.

After sharing her notes with the doctor, she wrote, "He states patient is to have routine blood pressure screenings at the clinic and an appointment has been scheduled for December 9th and Dr. E.M will review this information at that time with patient. Patient has been notified, and she is in agreement with this."

On December 9th, I had another doctor visit, my husband, Bob, came with me. I figured his coroboration of what I was telling the doctor might help.

The doctor wrote, "The patient is here with her husband today. She went on a bus ride to Missouri and had an exacerbation of her usual symptoms, including diarrhea, her hands being numb and tingly, pricking sensations all over, and sharp sensations that she likens to worms crawling under her skin. She also had achiness and malaise. She felt immediately better after starting the Keflex. She has been using eye ointments, despite the normal culture done by her eye doctor, Dr. H. These are apparently a sulfa and another type of antibiotic. She still experiences some discharge of a thick mucous out of her eyes every day. Again, she is insistent she is infected with a parasitic organism called *Capillaria aerophila* (or something similar)."

After the usual physical examination, he wrote: "The oral pharynx is normal. The chest is clear to auscultation. The abdominal exam is without masses. The skin exam is essentially normal. She has a few scattered cherry hemangiomas.

His assessment was, "Diffuse illness. We have essentially zero evidence for a parasitic or Helminth infection. However, after much consideration, I think that we're going to get nowhere unless we try some empiric treatment for this infection. I again emphasized the odds of her having this infection were in the range of one in a million. We looked into the medicine Albendazole, which is the recommended treatment for *Capillaria*. It appears to be safe, but allergic reactions can happen with any medications, and I did discuss this at length with the patient and her husband. The patient is very eager to proceed with therapy. We'll treat her with Albendazole for fourteen days, and then discontinue it for fourteen days. This pattern is to be repeated for a total of three cycles. The patient is to call me at the first sign of any allergic reaction.

"I am concerned about treating her irresponsibly, but I do think that to get her to understand her condition, this has to be done. If she is no better after this treatment, we'll discuss with her the possibility of delusion. I am quite concerned about her and want to do everything I can to help her. She agrees to proceed as we have planned. I will prescribe no other empiric therapy.

"For her hypothyroidism, she should have her TSH checked in approximately two months." Dr. E.M

"And goodness is the harvest that is produced from the seeds the peacemakers plant in peace."   James 3:18, Good News Bible.

I am so relieved that I finally will be treated for what all my research is pointing to as the cause of my bizarre symptoms. This has been an uphill climb. I am so grateful that my doctor is willing to try to treat me even though I have no diagnosis. *Thank you, Jesus.*

Whenever I started on a new antibiotic, I felt quite a bit better with a very predictable screech to a halt shortly after I completed it. There has to be some logical reason for this.

I was eager to start on the anti-parasite medication Albendazole that the *Oxford Companion* doctor suggested and my doctor finally wrote a prescription for. If Albendazole was to cure a possible parasite infection it cannot do the job on a short-term basis. There was a huge sense of relief that I could finally try something besides empirical antibiotics.

Finally things looked brighter.

But shortly after I started the Albendazole, I noticed the usual exacerbation of symptoms. Then a minor miracle happened, I actually felt lots, lots better except for my eyes. The dark exudate continued to plague me with intermittent sharp pains throughout my body and considerable diarrhea. But the miracle was that the worst of the systemic symptoms abated. I was so happy and I felt confident that finally the right medication had been prescribed, and I could get my life back. After all that unfolded since July, though, I was heavily skeptical. And rightly so. After the Albendazole was discontinued, many of my original symptoms returned.

But our lives continued. We joyfully were looking forward to the births of two grandbabies. While I was overjoyed with being a grandma, I was very concerned I might be contagious. All my doctors said I was not, but I still worried. I used anti-bacterial soaps and good hand washing. Thank heavens no members of our family or any of our friends contracted this thing.

This roller coaster was getting harder to stay on. The "well" me worked, socialized and participated in the usual family activities. The "sick" me fought an unseen monster that I felt I could tell no one about except my husband, Bob. When asked, I simply said I had an undiagnosed auto-immune disease, but I was getting better.

How I wished that were true. I was worried that, if left undiagnosed, a much more serious medical condition would soon follow. I, in my weakened condition, would be unable to fight it. It was starting to look like a life-and-death struggle.

In between doctor visits my mind raced with the what ifs.

At this point I had more questions than answers. I was determined to leave no stone unturned. And I am repeating all this here just in the slim chance someone somewhere will connect the dots. After all there are still a large number of very sick people out there with similar symptoms that need to get a diagnosis and help.

My doctor did not respond to this possibility or the others I had. I hesitated asking too many questions for fear I would be labeled delusional, but I had many, many questions. I just refused to give up as I knew there had to be an answer somewhere. I couldn't possibly be the only one ever to have these weird symptoms. Somewhere some place this must have been documented before.

Why did I get somewhat better on an antibiotic? Why couldn't doctors see my history of getting bit by something, and then developing large red sores on my torso, abdomen, and legs and connect this to a disease? Why couldn't doctors find a disease that included bite-like sensations followed by tiny red pupae especially on my ears? I HAVE SYMPTOMS! Why couldn't doctors see the possible connection between our sick dog and my symptoms? I explained that *Capillaria aerophilla* was found in Lacey's stool. I researched *Capillaria* and found that it is very rare but can be transferred to humans. Could that be what happened? If I could see this, why couldn't any medical professional?

My eye doctor's notes included this: "Painful headache, eyes mattery at night (awakens her at night). Concerned about redness and how long the problem is going on. On Tobradex ointment and sulfa—used three tubes."

On January 3rd, 1997, I contacted the Internal Medicine office. The nurse recorded this note: "Dr. E.M. asks if alkaline phosphatase and SGOT be scheduled. Appointment secretary will schedule necessary needed labs.

Ten days later I called the office, and the nurse's notes were: "Patient called questioning if follow-up thyroid testing needs to be done and Dr. E.M. states that this can be scheduled in February. Also states that she has volunteered for a skin sensation study in Minneapolis. Also questioning if records from the U of M Hospital have been sent to Clinic. These have not reached clinic, are not in patient's chart, and message has been left for patient at her home in regard to this with message to call if she has further concerns."

Regarding the skin sensation study, I had seen an ad in our newspaper entitled, "Bug biting, crawling, itching symptoms?" and gave a phone number.

I called out of curiosity. A Dr. Bart Gavin from the resident program at the university (Diehl Hall) was doing this research, and the psychiatry department was working in co-ordination with the dermatology department. When I briefly told them my situation, they asked if I was on an anti-psychotic drug. When I said no, they said I couldn't be considered for the study. I was left wondering what prompted the study and wondered what the results might have been. This could have been a black hole I wanted no part of. If I had agreed to take the Minnesota Multiphasic test months ago, it was entirely possible I would be on anti-psychotic drugs already, trapped in a cycle of side effects and labeling and a further spiraling down of my health with possibly lethal consequences. How many people got trapped that way, I would never know but it was terribly sad and, in my opinion, even could be categorized unethical.

On January 16th, I was working through a busy day, and it was nice to feel fairly normal. This level of symptoms I could almost live with. Was the Albendazole possibly working?

I had a visit with Dr. E.M., Internal Medicine specialist. He wrote: "Fifty-five-year-old woman here to see me in follow up for a multisystem illness. We had treated her with Albendazole for the very scant possibility that she had a parasitic disease. Karen herself feels that this was certainly the diagnosis and has noted sustained, but clear improvement over the last month. She has completed two two-week courses of Albendazole separated by two weeks. She has one course left. She notes no side effects from this. She states that the blackish discharge from her eyes is much better but still persistent. She also noted some generalized decrease in her visual acuity. She has a follow-up appointment scheduled with her eye doctor, Dr. H. She has occasional twinging pains, mostly around her eyes and her face. Her diarrhea has largely resolved. During this time she has also maintained her Synthroid dose. She is approximately six weeks now from initiation of treatment. On examination, her eyes appear normal. There is no discharge that I can identify. Oropharynx is normal. Chest is clear to auscultation."

His assessment was, "Karen is quite pleased with her progress. I am skeptical about the possibility of a parasitic infection, yet we will not do any more empiric treatment. She mentioned possible ASACOL for intermittent diarrhea, but I would prefer she see GI before we prescribe this. I certainly think some of her improvement could be due to hypothyroidism, and we will recheck a TSH to see if it is in the therapeutic level. I will see her again in three months. Her SGOT and alk phos are normal today."

Because Dr. E.M. had prescribed Albendazole on December 9th, 1996, and the treatment was to include fourteen days on and fourteen days off the medication, to be repeated for three cycles, this should have continued until March 9th, but on January 16th the treatment was stopped. When I asked Dr. M to continue the Albendazole, he declined. Had I been on it long enough to do any good long term?

On February 6th, I had an office visit with Dr. H., a gastroenterologist. His notes identified the reason for the visit: "Abdominal cramps and diarrhea. This pleasant fifty-four-year-old female is seen today at the request of her primary care provider, Dr. E.M. This patient has been experiencing a very unusual process that is well documented by Dr. E.M. in his notes. Briefly, the patient has felt that she picked up an unusual parasite from her dog.

"Exam reveals a pleasant lady in no acute distress. Vital signs are unremarkable. Weight is stable. Currently, skin is free of any rashes or abnormalities. Nodes-negative. Chest-clear. Abdomen-soft, scaphoid and free of any focal tenderness, masses or heptosplenomegaly. Bowel sounds are normal.

"I am really at a loss to explain the patient's recent systemic illness. It appears to have resolved with the current empiric therapy, which we are all grateful for. I have explained to her that the remaining irregularity in her bowel pattern most likely are secondary to motility dysfunction. She has not been using any fiber supplementation. I have informed her that an increase of fiber in her GI tract will probably bring about resolution of these minimal dysmotility symptoms. I do not feel that she requires any further investigations and/or endoscopic studies; she is comfortable with this assessment.

"1. Utilize fiber supplement—Citrucel one tablespoon one to two times per day. I have recommended she continue this long-term.

"2. The patient will continue follow-up with Dr. E.M. for primary care. I will see her on a prn basis."

I was pleased that all my gastric turmoil did not appear to have caused any life threatening disease at this point. I started on the Citrucel as prescribed and hoped for the best. But I was very concerned that my symptoms would return as I was not being allowed to continue on the Albendazole, which I felt had helped me considerably. I was concerned that the length of time I took this medication would be insufficient to be therapeutic.

Oh, happy day! In February, Bob and I welcomed the birth of our first grandchild, precious Paige, born to our youngest son and his beautiful wife. She was a gorgeous, perfect baby. I was overjoyed but this darling child's birth made me more determined than ever to get totally well so I could love and care for her as grandmas want to do. I wanted so badly to hug and squeeze her but I just couldn't be sure I wasn't contagious, so kept my distance. When I held her I was very careful not to get too close to her face and washed my hands multiple times. This is not a good situation for a brand new Grandma to find herself in. It saddened me a great deal.

On March 7th, I called Dr. E.M. He had these notes: "Patient called yesterday to clarify when her next TSH level is to be drawn, and I have informed her it is scheduled for March 25th. Also patient complaining that she is having lots of eye fluttering and mattering waking her up at night. She also states she has a prickly pinch feeling on her skin. She doesn't know if it is internal, especially right under the skin. She states mostly this occurs in the back of her head as well as her waist, but at times will occur all over her body. She says that this feeling happens approximately every hour. Other than that, she states she is feeling quite well. Also has seen her eye doctor, Dr. H., in regard to the infection with her eyes. Treatment did not help."

Dr. E.M.'s nurse states, "If patient continues to have problems with her eyes, he would suggest her again seeing Dr. H. or using some over-the-counter lubricating drops. In speaking with patient, she states that she has recently seen Dr. H. and has been using lubricating drops for approximately two months and will call if she has any further concerns. Also, patient this morning upon return phone call is asking Dr. E.M. to call her. She says she has a concern that she would like to share with him. I have informed patient, Dr. E.M. is not in the office today and requests that he call her back on March 10th.

Sadly my sick days were back. Many symptoms have returned; which was very agonizing to say the least. I had been concerned that my doctor would not let me complete the three cycles of Albendazole and now fear that my earlier symptoms have returned because of the aborted course of treatment.

I decided I had to start thinking out of the box. I had tried for over nine months working with the medical community and felt I was sliding back into the throes of this totally unpredictable illness.

If the Albendazole had worked so well (albeit temporarily), would another anti-parasitic work as well? I decided to try Piperazine tablets and hope for the best. I must confess I was scared but determined. I needed to get well however I could. After all I had a new grandbaby I wanted to enjoy. The medical community either would not or could not do much for me anymore. At this point the devil I knew was worse than the possible side effects I might encounter.

I took Piperazine from March 8th to 24th. After the Piperazine cycle, my symptoms exacerbated to a higher level. After first getting some relief, perhaps I needed to have repeated the original applications, but I was afraid to do so.

I noticed considerable redness and matting of my eyes. There was white, stringy matter in my mouth. The severe twitching in and around my eyes had greatly decreased, but I continued to get sharp punches in back of the head.

"Make sure you obey the Law that Moses commanded you. Love the Lord your God, do His will, obey His commandments, be faithful to Him, and serve Him with all your heart and soul."   Joshua 22:5 Good News Bible

Oh, how very hard it is to see that a cure was not yet to be. I especially was dismayed that I was now so weak and was experiencing brain fog. Having lived in our town all my life, I knew basic roads and directions quite well. One day I found myself totally unable to navigate a road I had traveled many times. I stopped the car dead near some railroad tracks to get my bearings, and I honestly felt I was just going to cry. But instead, I just sat in my car numb with nothing.

By the middle of March, my symptoms were increasing. The filamentous matter observed during the night in my mouth woke me up. I gargled, but it stuck to my tongue. Examination showed string-like whitish, inch-long pieces of something. But what?

Alarmed, I decided to call Dr. E.M. again and ask if he could order lab specs taken of this whitish matter. I wanted it to be observed under a microscope. I was also very concerned that I might be contagious to my new grandbaby. I asked if he would consider represcribing Albendazole. It had worked the best of anything else, and so many of my symptoms were returning. An appointment was made for March 24th, 1997.

At that visit, Dr. E.M. again took my history: "Karen Ament is a fifty-five-year-old woman who returns for a routine visit. She has had some increasing symptoms recently that she would like to discuss with me. She has had a nagging illness for the last year, which has manifested in a variety of symptoms. She states that she is much better than she was before with taking the Albendazole, and is "not systemically" ill now. She does not have the diarrhea and fatigue she had previously. She does, however, have the following symptoms—a stringy, white mucus discharge in her mouth and tongue; a red rash around her waist area that prickles and is widely distributed; severe itching in her scalp; a dark, mucus-like exudate from her eyes that she is most concerned about; a stiff neck; and an earache. She also describes some black-and-blue marks that appear to be bruises. Karen has read extensively about her symptoms and wonders if she could have *Cryptococcus neoformans*. She is also worried about being with her grandchild and making her sick. On examination, she appears discouraged. Her vital signs are normal. Her eyes appear normal. There is no exudate and there is no conjunctiva inflammation. Her mouth appears normal.

Her neck is supple. There is no lymphadenopathy. The chest is clear to auscultation. She has some pinpoint, scattered, scabbed lesions that are consistent with excoriation. The heart exam is normal. The abdomen is normal. She does have some bruises that are in the blue-to-yellow stage over her anterior thighs. These are not extensive. There is no lymphadenopathy in her groin or axillae. Her lower extremities are normal."

On reading these notes, I almost had to laugh when I read, "she appears discouraged." Discouraged is putting it mildly! Nine months of living a nightmare could easily discourage most people. Thank heavens I did not know that I would have almost four more years of this scenario.

"The Lord said, 'I will go with you, and I will give you victory.'"
Exodus 33:14 Good News Bible

Even in the darkest times of discouragement I felt His presence, and I felt at rest in His care. "Jesus help me" was my mantra.

After the laboratory studies, Dr. E.M. got back to me. "Her CBC, Eosinophil count, urinalysis, glucose, and chem panel are pending. A TSH was 0.58 recently, which is in the therapeutic range," he wrote, and added this assessment: "Multisystem illness. Again Karen is concerned about this, although she feels she is better than she has been. My impression is that she feels one infectious agent is causing her symptoms. Again, we discussed the importance of not launching on a battery of tests, although she states, 'I would have any test, including a spinal tap, to find out what is wrong with me.' We need to monitor her symptoms at regular intervals and use medical logic to dictate and evaluate. At this point, I don't see any evidence for an infectious agent. She did not focus on worms as being the source of her problem today. I stated that she could bring in some samples of the exudate, and we would examine those under the microscope. Again, I have not brought up the possibility of parasitosis as being an etiology for her illness, although this is still possible. She is not fixated exclusively on worms or parasites. I have advised her that she meet with me every six weeks."

By the end of the month, I was at my wits end. I had had a really bad night. Fluttering of my eyes and continuous discharge and matting. Severe insomnia. I decided I would have to call my doctor and ask for another referral to Eye Surgeons and Physicians. Or anyone else that could help me.

When I called on the 31st, the nurse wrote: "This patient calls in stating she needs to talk to Dr. E.M. today." After she spoke to him, she wrote, "He requests that I return a phone call to the patient and find out what the signs and symptoms are that she is experiencing. I placed a call to patient and her current signs and symptoms are that she'd had a bad weekend. She has a lot of mattering bilateral discharge. She requests another referral to see her eye specialist Dr. H. Eyes have been real fluttery with a lot of activity around the eyes. She has a decreased amount of sleep. This is causing her to feel very fatigued. I reviewed all of this with Dr. E.M. and he suggests that patient has a visit with Dr. J. at the Eye Surgeons and Physicians. He has okayed two visits. The diagnosis for this would be conjunctivitis. (I did fill out the referral procedure and will hand this to nurse for her to follow up on.) Patient was notified of the referral to see Dr. J as associate of Dr. H.

I submitted a note previous to this doctor visit that included the following:

Eye symptoms:

1. Dark, stringy, mucousy matter (needs to be wiped out of corners of eyes often eight to twelve times/day and also at night and especially in morning. Itching and twitching.

2. Insomnia due to fluttering of eyes during night—it wakes me up and then hard to get back to sleep.

3. Matting—sometimes it's hard to open my eyes. In the morning I notice a whitish, crusty matter around eyes.

4. Sometimes black dark matter is found clinging to white of eyes.

Again any of these individual symptoms could be easily ignored, but taken in a larger context seem to point to a systemic illness with a cause and explanation and a diagnosis.

Chapter Seven

Medical Meandering
and Miscellany

APRIL BEGAN, AND I STARTED to realize that being sick this long was very unhealthy. All my adult life, I had only taken a multi-vitamin pill, but now I started to think I needed antioxidants to help protect cells from damage caused by free radicals and whatever else I had going on. They also protected biological membranes found in nerves, muscles, and the cardiovascular system. I started taking over-the-counter sleep aids—Melatonin and Valerian. They did help some. I added garlic, vitamin E, licorice root, a probiotic, vitamin C, calcium, L-Cysteine, and vitamin A.

I guess I should have rejoiced as I now had a diagnosis of sorts—conjunctivitis, blepharitis, and dry-eye, along with hypothyroidism. It felt good going in to a doctor armed with a real diagnosis. But I totally knew this was a side result of my original disease, which remained undiagnosed. But my eyes were a concern, and I knew I again needed to see a doctor for my eye symptoms. Maybe something would click from this visit towards the cause of my eye symptoms.

I had two visits with Dr. J., on April 2nd and 4th. After the first visit, Dr. J. noted, "Describes symptoms of mattering in a.m.- itchy, achy, more blurry eyes." Then, on the 4th, she added, "Seeing Dr. E.M.'s patient—was ill July 20th through December. Dr. not sure what it was. Dark, stringy, mucous eyes for seven months. Eyes are matted and shut in morning. Refresh plus q hour helps, but she wakes up during night with sticky eyes, make up has been changed twice."

I then had a follow-up visit with Dr. J. on the 7th. She prescribed

Erythromycin ointment and to discard all mascara. I did this and used the ointment with no improvement at all. Another dead end.

"But I know there is someone in Heaven who will come at last to my defense."
Job 19:25 Good News Bible.

Hope springs eternal.

I started to wonder if perhaps Lymes was still a possibility. Many of my symptoms matched, but many did not. Some first-stage symptoms matched mine—malaise, arthralgia (pain in joints), inflammation, and conjunctivitis. The second phase symptoms matched my later stage symptoms very closely.

1. Neurologic and cardiac problems—high BP and racing heart, tingling.

2. Cranial nerve palpitations—almost constant drilling in the back of my head

3. Optic neuropathy and eye disease

Dr. W.T. Harvey, P. Salvato, Diversified Medical Practices, Houston, Texas, issued a Medical Hypotheses entitled "Lyme disease": ancient engine of an unrecognized borreliosis pandemic? His summary is as follows:

> Unexpectedly we have found large numbers of chronically ill Borrelia burgdorferi PCR—and seropositive patients in Houston, Texas, a zoonotically "non-endemic" area. In order to understand this finding prior to sufficient data availability, we chose to examine critically currently accepted but troublesome "Lyme disease" concepts. Our method was to analyze each foundation "Lyme disease" premise within the context of available medical and veterinary literature, then to reconstruct the disease model consistent with the preponderance of that data. We find the present conceptualization of the illness seriously truncated, with a high likelihood of two distinct but connected forms of human *B. burgdorferi* infection. The yet-unrecognized form appears to have a broader clinical presentation, wider geographic distribution, and vastly greater prevalence. We conclude that "Lyme disease" currently acknowledges only its zoonosis arm and is a limited conceptualization of

a far more pervasive and unrecognized infection state that must be considered a global epidemic. (2003 Elesvier Science Ltd.)

I have included this data because of the similarity of symptoms between what I was experiencing compared to typical end Lyme's symptoms. Is there any connection in any way?

By mid-April, my ever changing daily symptoms are: Neck ache, headache, backache, dull ear ache, eyes sore, eyes twitching, eye exudate (dark), drilling (intermittent) back of head, joint pain, knees and hips, and legs weak.

There seemed to be enough matches that I called Dr. E.M. to discuss again. The nurse made notes: "Patient called this morning just questioning if she was ever tested for Lyme disease, states when she initially started with the problems, that she had started with large welts on her abdomen and torso that resembled pictures that she has seen in regard to Lyme disease. States she is doing much better. Continues to have eye mattering. Sharp pinches (?) on her body are almost gone.

I didn't like what I felt was some manner of disconnect on my conveying what I was experiencing. The nurse had said, "States she is doing much better." She should have stated, "Many original symptoms abated but others are now present."

"Lyme titer was drawn on November twenty first and was non-reactive. This information relayed back to patient. She is requesting to speak with Dr. E.M. States she now feels she has second-stage Lyme disease and knows that the blood test at times may be false. Office visit has been scheduled with Dr. E.M. for further discussion.

More questioning few answers. On the 16th, I decided to write a letter to Dr. E.M. "Because I am still having symptoms and my initial episode started with observance of tiny black bugs with subsequent circular red sores following sometime after and the close similarity of the symptoms of Lymes and what is currently happening to me I wanted to ask you if you could definitely rule out Lymes. I understand my blood test for Lymes was negative on November 21st, 1996, but also I am aware that false negatives are common. These are the symptoms of Lymes that I obtained from a medical resource book from the U of M.

First Phase:
* Regional lymphadenopathy, malaise, fever, headaches, myalgia, arthralgia, conjunctivitis.
Second Phase:
* Neurologic and cardiac problems, cranial nerve palsy, optic neuropathy, uveitis—inflammation of uvea, choroiditis—inflammation of the choroid.

After my months of being so sick subsided somewhat, I am now experiencing these symptoms observed and reported on April 15th: Neck ache, headache, backache, dull ear ache, eyes sore, eyes twitching —often especially at night—eye exudate (dark), drilling to back of head (intermittent), joint pain in my knees and hips, legs weak.

What can be causing these symptoms? I had none of these before July of 1996.

P.S. Copy to eye doctor

P.P.S. List of medications taken: Amoxicillin, Bactrim, Erythromycin, Cipro, Flagyl and Albendazol. Eye ointments prescribed: Metimyd OP, Tobradex, and Erythromycin.

On April 16th I had an appointment with the eye doctor, Dr. J. She discontinued the erythromycin ointment and ordered acetycysteine and warm compresses. It helped a little, but the black stringy substance is still present.

By the 19th, I was starting to feel a little better but my eyes were still a problem. At times the black mucous substance feels like course sand.

April 24th, Bob and I are happily anticipating the birth of our second grandchild to arrive any day. I do so want to be healthy so I can enjoy this baby and also my first grandbaby. Also on that day, I saw Dr. E.M. He wrote: " Karen Ament is seen in follow up. Startlingly, she says, 'I feel great.' She states that last weekend she woke up and felt like her old self. She has had five days of this. Before that, she was having many symptoms, which are outlined in her note to me, including arthralgias, fatigue, tingling pains, headaches, neck ache, and backache, as well as her continuing eye symptoms. She is on a lot of complementary therapies, including shark cartilage, garlic, Vitamin E, calcium, and other antioxidants. She is working with eye doctor Dr. J. as well. She is getting Erythromycin ointment and Refresh drops. On examination, her eyes appear normal. There is no discharge and there is no redness. At this point, Karen is only asking for a Lyme titer rechecks, which was negative in November. It is conceivable that she could have the condition and have been partially cured with antibiotics, leading to a negative antibody response. I agreed to another serologic test. Certainly, her symptoms are not in any way classic for Lyme disease. If she had a positive titer, we would have to more consider Western blot testing. If this is negative, I think she would be satisfied with this. She will continue to see her eye doctor Dr. J. regarding her eye symptoms."

04/29/97

Oh, happy day. In the midst of so much confusion, worry and sickness, our second grandbaby, Nicholas, was born the end of April to our daughter and son-in-law. He was a perfect, handsome, beautiful baby, and we were so happy to welcome him to our family. Mom and baby (and Dad) were doing well.

My daughter called me at work several hours before she went to the hospital, and I tried to concentrate but couldn't, so I drove seventy miles to the hospital and waited in the adjoining waiting room for our first grandson's arrival. He arrived at 5:57 p.m. Bob and all the rest of our immediate family all joined us in the hospital to congratulate the proud parents and marvel at the perfection of this new baby boy.

I now had two grandbabies, and I knew I needed to double up my efforts to get well so I could spend more time with them. With all the cleansings and anti-parasitic treatments I had taken, I felt I was not contagious, but I still had bothersome lingering symptoms. My doctors all said I was not contagious, but I could not risk even the slightest possibility so was extremely careful around my grandbabies.

Actually it broke my heart.

My next appointment with Dr. J. seemed almost a non sequitur. On May 7th, all she wrote was "Eyes still mattering and itching. Fluttering gone."

Later that month, on the 22nd, I had a very sad day. My father died unexpectedly at the hospital of a heart attack at age eighty-three. He had been doctoring, but neither he nor we expected something like this to happen. He died in the emergency room with my sister Pauline and me with him. We had been planning a family reunion, and all five of us "kids" were looking forward to being together with Mom and Dad and assorted family members. Michael, Susanne, Pauline, and Jayne were coming home to celebrate; instead we all had to say goodbye to our dad. It was an emotional, trying time for all of us, and especially our mom. I did the eulogy for him at his Mass service. It was my final gift to him.

But life continued, and my situation sadly continued as well. I needed to spend a lot of time with my mother who needed comfort and help. She was still in her own home, but had a doggie to care for and considerable health problems. I never did tell her of my ongoing dilemma. It just felt better to concentrate on her needs. She would have been very troubled to know what I had going on and my resultant confusion and distress because of it.

"The winter is over; the rains have stopped; in the countryside the flowers are in bloom. This is the time for singing; the song of doves is heard in the fields."
Song of Songs 2:11-12 Good News Bible

Yes Spring is here. Praise the Lord.

I went to see Dr. J. on June 11th. I still had a black, stringy mucous substance frequently in in eyes. Sometimes it felt like sand. It matted during the night and early mornings. Dr. J. prescribed Albumin. I took this until June 15 and then needed to discontinue it due to an allergic reaction—red blotchy cheeks, a neck so stiff I could hardly move it, itchy face and right arm, and I also felt feverish. And that was after Dr. J.'s note, "Eyes not as sore. Still has discharge."

Also on the 15th, I woke up often during the night with a strong pulse. I could even feel the pulse beats in my fingers when holding an object. I noted puffiness below my left eye.

On the 18th, I woke up twice to exudate, stringy, mucousy, dark stuff in my eyes. The right eye had more than left eye. My neck continues to be stiff. On the 28th, I started on erythromycin eye ointment. The black, mucousy exudate in my eyes continues. It felt like sand in my eyes especially in the morning. It took lots of Q-tips to clear it out, and I'd use Refresh drops to get it all out. My eyes itched too, and my neck and skull towards my ears felt very stiff. I discontinued the erythromycin and started on acetylcysteine ten to four drops a day.

On June 30th, my eye doctor Dr. J. referred me to the University of Minnesota to see eye doctor Dr. H. (Department of Opthamology Corneal Specialist) Phillip Wangensteen Building on July 28th. My sister Sue, a nurse practitioner, would go with me. I planned to ask Dr. H. about any possibility of Retinoblastoma? Toxoplasm Parasite? Trichinella Parasite? Fusciolopsis? Were there any other parasites of the eye?

Dr. J. wrote: "Patient called. Having a lot of neck pain. Patient should see her primary care doctor. Did refer to the "U" to see Dr. H. Will send copy of records to patient."

My eyes itched in intervals throughout the day, sometimes it felt like squiggles as if something was actually moving. A dark mucous matter still formed often, sometimes apparent clinging to the white of the eye. I needed to wipe it out fifteen to twenty five times a day.

Looking back over almost one full year of this affliction, I tabulated medications I used. Some gave me initial relief but it would be years before I felt normal.

1. Cyproheptadine (Periactin)
2. Amoxicillin
3. Bactrim
4. Erythromicin

5. Cipro

6. Flagyl

7. Albendazole (Note: Dosage possibly less than required to cure a parasitic infection taken December 9, 1996 to January 16, 1997.

8. Eye Medications—Muro ointment three to four times a day, Erythromycin ointment, Tobradex ointment, Metimyd OP Sulfacetamide/Prednisone, Acetycysteine , Albumin ophthalmic drops, sty ointment (mercuric acid), continuous use of Refresh lubricant drops and hot packs often.

9. Benadryl cream

10. Benadryl tablets

11. Lotrimin fungal cream

12. Cortizone spray

13. Triamcinalon 0.1 %(corticosteroid cream)

14. Clarinex tablets (anti-histamine)

15. Anti-biotic cream

On July 25th, I had the scheduled appointment with Dr. H. My nurse practitioner sister Sue accompanied me. The doctor was able to observe:

1. Conjunctivitis

2. Conjunctiva cysts (they may be caused by allergy problems, trauma, infection, or disrupted glands).

3. Dry eye; Laser surgery may be needed. Note my eye doctor will review notes from U and will try to use a plug (temporary) to see if this helps before laser surgery.

Dr. H. sent this letter to my eye doctor with a copy to my medical doctor:

University of Minnesota   August 1, 1997
Department of Ophthalmology
Box 493, 420 Delaware Street, S.E.
Minneapolis, MN. 55455-0501
RE: Karen Ament

Dear Dr. J.,

Thank you for referring the above patient who was examined in our clinic on July 28, 1997. As you recall, this 54 year old woman has an approximate one year history of persistent itching, burning and mattering of both eyes which began approximately six weeks after an apparent episode of systemic parasitic infection. She has been on various topical therapies including Mkuro 128, vitamin A, erythromycin and acetylcysteine. These have resulted in a variable to minimal response. Current medications include Synthroid. She was on a course of Flagyl in November and Albendazole middle of December to middle of January.

On examination, visual acuity without correction is 20/20 in the right eye and 20/20 in the left eye. With appropriate reading correction, she is able to read the j line on the near card. Pupils are normal as are visual fields to confrontation and extra ocular movements. Slit lamp examination reveals bilateral temporal limbal subconjunctival concretions. This is not associated with any localized conjunctival or episcleral injection. She demonstrates no evidence of inflammation in the anterior chamber, and a slight anterior capsular opacity in the right eye. Schirmer's testing without anesthesia for five minutes reveals 13 mm of tear production in the right eye and 10 mm in the left. Staining of the ocular surface with Rose Bengal reveals a few spots of inferior punctate staining at the 6:00 position and larger areas of conjunctival staining which measure approximately 1.5 x 1 cm in the inferior bulbar conjunctiva OU. A fundus examination reveals no posterior pole abnormality. Cup to disc ratios are approximately 0.5 OU and symmetric.

IMPRESSION:
Ms. Ament suffers from persistent complaints of itchiness, burning and mattering of both eyes for approximately one year. Schirmer's testing and Rose Bengal staining patterns of the ocular surface are highly suggestive of keratoconjunctivitis sicca. Specifically, there is no intense papillary or follicular conjunctival reaction or other suggestion of acute or chronic infectious process.

PLAN:
We have suggested to Ms. Ament to continue her use of non-preserved artificial tear preparations every one to

two hours and have recommended argon laser punctual occlusion for relief of her symptoms of keratoconjunctivitis sicca. She is considering these options, and will return to us as necessary for argon laser punctaplasty.
Thank you for referring this interesting patient to our clinic.
Sincerely,
Dr. H., M.D.
Professor
Director, Cornea and External Disease Service

On August 12th, I had an appointment with Dr. J. He wrote, "She inserted temporary plugs into my eyes to retain my tears better. Said cysts are not likely to be caused by parasites. (I had asked her). Next step—laser if this helps—permanent but can be reversed." His further note: "Two month check. Chronic conjunctivitis. Col. Punctual plugs today. Rx Refresh q. one half hour."

The next day I called my eye doctor and had a conversation. Dr. J. wrote, "Eyes feel a lot better. Still mattery but not as dry. When she wipes eyes will that shift the plugs? Getting bruises on legs from autoimmune."

Chapter Eight

Into the World
of Natural Healing

I MAGINE HAVING TO TALK to my eye doctor about bruises on my legs! I was really getting desperate and hoping against hope that someone, anyone, would just connect the dots, but perhaps to expect my eye doctor to do this was ridiculous.

After this appointment I decided I needed to move out of the standard medical box and be open to additional alternative medicine. However, I had no idea how to start or who to see or what to do. I had tried odds and ends of herbals and cleansings, but knew I needed to move into a definite plan using naturopathic experts' advice.

I also knew—was fully convinced even if the medical doctors weren't—that I had contracted something awful in the middle of July 1996. I had a long list of physical symptoms to prove it. I was very disappointed that medical doctors discounted most of my symptoms because they didn't know what I had. They slipped so easily into believing I had some mental illness. I slipped further and further until I was barely functioning and finally realized medical doctors were not able to help me. I was not going to get relief from them. I was not angry with the medical experts, but I was adamant that other people caught in the same dilemma should feel free to step outside the medical box as I did and get well. I also started pondering how to present my unusual data in hopes that someone somewhere could use my sequence of events and identify it with others having similar experiences.

"God helps those who help themselves" came to mind.

I was now armed with a courage I never thought I had, never imagined I would need. I opened up our Yellow Pages and found a health food store. I had never been in one before as I thought they sold nothing but quack items or certainly nothing that could be of much help to anyone. I thought they were just a waste of money. We should be able to get all our nutrients through the food we eat. Right?

I had no idea even what to look for or to ask for. The clerk (Joanie) asked me what I needed. I said I was just looking. A small bookshelf stood against one wall, and there were a few shelves loaded with bottles with strange names. The bookshelf caught my eye, and I perused the titles. None seemed to capture any of my problems. I did feel that my situation was parasitic in origin, so asked Joanie if she had anything that might include that. She said she did not but showed me a book, *The Cure for All Cancers* by Hulda Regehr Clark, Ph.D., N.D. The cover included the following: "Including over 100 Case Histories of Persons cured . . . Plus two revolutionary electronic circuits, one to diagnose and monitor progress, the other to zap parasites and bacteria."

I glanced over my shoulder as I read the back cover and hoped no one I knew saw me reading this book. I perused it to discover that: Dr. Clark was an independent research scientist. She began her studies in biology at the University of Saskatchewan, Canada, where she was awarded the Bachelor of Arts, Magna Cum Laude, and Master of Arts-with High Honors. After two years of study at McGill University, she attended the University of Minnesota, studying biophysics and cell physiology. She received a Doctorate degree in physiology in 1958. In 1979 she left government-funded research and began private consulting on a full-time basis. Six years later she discovered an electronic technique for scanning the human body.

This scientist traveled a "road less traveled" when she conducted research out of the main stream and then followed it up with case histories and then a book. I paged through her book and found that almost everything looked foreign to me. The whole concept she raised and the methods she used to assess her patients were not mainstream to say the least. If I were not so sick, I would never have purchased the book. But I was and I bought it.

The author had impressive credentials. I was surprised that a woman of this stature would write such an unconventional book, but I knew I needed to read it.

Okay, this would be my start. I had to step out of my comfort zone anyway, so why not go for a far-out author's discovery? I headed home with the book and started dinner, which was a hurried affair as I could not put this book down. I read it cover to cover in one sitting, reading late into the night. I don't even remember if I ate dinner.

Dr. Clark's foreword intrigued me greatly. "Cancer Can Now Be Cured, Not Just Treated."

Of course I did not have cancer, but her references to parasitic involvement in many diseases intrigued me. I still felt strongly that there was a causative agent involved with my myriad of symptoms.

"We are not accustomed to thinking about a cure for cancer," she wrote. "We think of remission as the only possibility. But this book is not about remission. It is about a cure. This is possible because in 1990 I discovered the true cause of cancer. The cause is a certain parasite, for which I have found evidence in every cancer case regardless of the type of cancer. So lung cancer is not caused by smoking, colon cancer is not caused by a low-roughage diet, breast cancer is not caused by a fatty diet, retinal blastoma is not caused by a rare gene, and pancreatic cancer is not caused by alcohol consumption. Although these are all contributing factors, they are not *the* cause. Once the true cause was found, the cure became obvious. But would it work? I set a goal of 100 cases to be cured of cancer before publishing my findings. That mark was passed in December 1992. The discovery of the cause and cure of all cancers has stood the test of time and here it is!"

Was this absolutely ridiculous talk? If a cause and cure for cancer had been found why had no medical journals with research picked this up. What is this talk about cancer curing and electricity—zapping parasites? I should return this book in the morning. I then started to read it just a little bit more. I thought this woman with appropriate degrees and research credentials had gone off her rocker. Really smart people can be crazy too, right? But what if she were right—even a little? And what if I tried some of her recipes and got well? What did I care if they were far out? I needed relief at any cost. And, besides, I did not have cancer, not yet anyway. However, I was starting to feel I might succumb eventually if I couldn't figure this thing out. Obviously I not only continued but finished the book and made a list of what products to buy right away and started doing what Dr. Clark recommended. What could it hurt anyway?

Another trip to Inez Health Food Store to purchase the ingredients for the Parasite Killing Program.

I wanted to thoroughly research the herbs Dr. Clark recommended in her book, so I also purchased a copy of *PDR for Herbal Medicines*, first edition. The 1999 *PDR for Herbal Medicine* touted, "the most comprehensive prescribing reference of its kind is based upon the work conducted by renowned botanist, Joerg Gruenwald, Ph.D. and the German Federal Authority's Commission E, the governmental body widely recognized as having conducted the most authoritative evaluation of herbs in the world. Entries include the pharmacological effects of each plant, applicable precautions, warning, interactions and contraindications, administration and dosages, adverse reactions and overdose data, plus much more."

This book became my bible of sorts when deciding what herbals to use during my recovery.

Dr. Clark's main herbal program included the following, and the PDR reported these statistics:

1. Black Walnut Hull tincture extra strength. EFFECTS: The main active principles are the tannins and juglon. There is an astringent effect because of the tannins. The antifungal effect comes from the juglon content and the essential oil. Externally, walnut is used for mild, superficial inflammation of the skin and excessive perspiration. Internally, the drug is used for gastrointestinal catarrh and as an anthelmintic (so-called blood purifier). No health hazards or side effects are known in conjunction with the proper administration of designated therapeutic dosages.

2. Wormwood capsules. In folk medicine, wormwood preparations are used internally for gastric insufficiency, intestinal atonia, gastritis, stomach-ache, liver disorders, bloating, anemia, irregular menstruation, intermittent fever, loss of appetite, and worm infestation. Externally the drug is applied for poorly healing wounds, ulcers, skin blotches, and insect bites. Continuous use is not advisable. INDICATIONS AND USAGE: Loss of appetite, dyspeptic complaints and liver and gall bladder complaints.

3. Cloves (I made my own per Dr. Clark's instructions) EFFECTS: Clove is antiseptic, antibacterial, antifungal, antiviral, spasmolytic and a local anesthetic. INDICATIONS AND USAGE: Common cold, cough/bronchitis, dental analgesic, fevers and colds, inflammation of the mouth and pharynx, tendency to infection. No health hazards or side effects are known in conjunction with the proper administration of designated therapeutic dosages.

4. Ornithine (at bedtime for insomnia) Dr.Clark says, "Parasites produce a great deal of ammonia as their waste products, ammonia is their equivalent of urine and it is set free in our bodies by parasites in large amounts. Ammonia is very toxic, especially to the brain. I believe this causes insomnia and other sleep problems at night and anxiety by day. By taking ornithine at bedtime, you will sleep better. There are no side-effects. There is no interference with any other medication. There is no need to stop any treatment that a clinical doctor or alternative therapist has started you on."

5. Niacinamide Helps detoxify the alcohol in the tincture.

I decided to start with an intense program because I felt I had no time to lose. I wanted to hit my affliction with the strongest prescription recommended, a one-time treatment to be followed by the regular routine.

I started with: (per Dr. Clark's suggestions)

  Eight teaspoons of black walnut tincture

  Three 500 mg niacin amide tablets

  Rested one hour and repeated

I did not use the Zapper as I had not sent for it yet.

I soon felt light-headed and my head and eye area ached much more than usual. I had considerable tingling sensations around my nose especially. And a stiff neck. Aching of upper my arms, especially strong at my armpits and forearm areas. I had chills and felt feverish. Multi stools. Nausea. A headache continued across my forehead and eye sockets. My legs were weak, and I had a severe ache in my right shoulder. I was sick all day—really sick—but I toughed it out.

As before when I started an antibiotic or especially the Albendazole, I got a lot worse before I got any better but this program was bad in spades—Whew what a trip!

I felt as if I was on a giant roller coaster as the zigs and zags and symptoms raged continuously. My head felt like it might explode, my neck was very stiff, I had lots of black mucous in eyes, white mucous in my nose and throat. I felt gassy, had a rumbling tummy and ached all over. What in the world was happening inside of my body? I could only imagine the fight of a lifetime going on. Somebody was going to win, and I hoped it would be me.

Dear Lord if this wasn't so ridiculous, I could ignore it. But how can I? I had no choice but to plow ahead into unchartered territory. Thinking of Jackie Gleason, I could only say, "And away we go!"

I then started the Maintenance Parasite Program. Dr. Clark said, "You are always picking up parasites! Parasites are everywhere around you! You get them from other people, your family, yourself, your home, your pets, undercooked meat, and undercooked dairy products."

Dr. Clark's Maintenance Parasite Program:
1. Black Walnut Hull Tincture Extra Strength: two teaspoons on an empty stomach, like before a meal or bedtime.
2. Wormwood capsules: seven capsules (with 200-300 mg wormwood each) once a day on an empty stomach.
3. Cloves: three capsules (500 mg each, or fill size 00capsules yourself) once a day on an empty stomach.
4. Take ornithine as needed.
(See Dr. Clark's instructions for additional information)

After twelve days of this cleanse, I woke up and actually felt better—a lot better. I truly felt this was the path I needed to take.

Because it took me a long time to get as sick as I was, I knew it would also be a long time before I got my health completely back.

My subsequent research led me to also add:

1. Red Clover Blossoms: Trifolium Piatense. Has antispasmodic and expectorant effects and also promotes the skin's healing process. Internally, Red Clover is used for coughs and respiratory conditions.

2. Grape Juice: *Vitus vinifera*. The flavonoid in the leaves has an anti-inflammatory and "phlebitis" effect. Grape preparations are used in venous diseases and blood circulation disorders. No health hazards or side effects are known in conjunction with the proper administration of designated therapeutic dosages.

3. Pumpkin Seeds: *CucurBita pepo*. In folk medicine, pumpkin seed is used for kidney inflammation, intestinal parasites, particularly tape worm and vulnary.

4. Golden Seal: *Hydrastis canadensis*. Used in homeopathic dilutions for internal administration and used externally on wounds and herpes labialis.

5. Milk Thistle: *Silybum marianum*. The drug is used for dyspeptic complaints, toxic liver damage, supportive treatments in chronic inflammatory liver disease and hepatic cirrhosis.

6. Licorice Root: *Glycyrrhiza glabra*. Used in the treatment of viral liver inflammation (also post-hepatital liver cirrhosis). The juice may work as an antiviral agent by means of interferon induction.

7. Acidophilus: Probiotic. Aids in maintaining healthy balance of intestinal flora.

8. Garlic: *Allium sativum*. In folk medicine, garlic is utilized internally for arteriosclerosis, high blood pressure, colds, coughs, whooping cough, and bronchitis. Garlic is also used for gastrointestinal ailments, particularly for digestive disorders with bloating and convulsive pain. Other uses include: menstrual pains, treatment of diabetes. Externally for corns, warts, calluses, otitis, muscle pain, neuralgia, arthritis and sciatica.

9. St. John's Wort: *Hypericum perforatum*. For anxiety, depressive moods, inflammation of the skin, blunt injuries, wounds, and burns.

I used these herbs according to directions on the labels and usually only took one bottle and discontinued it.

Data provided by: *The PDR for Herbal Medicines*, the Information Standard for Complementary Medicine. Section: Herbal Monographs.

Because I continued to feel so much better with Dr. Clark's recommendations but still was experiencing symptoms, I purchased another of her books, *The Cure for All Diseases*. I also read this book cover to cover. Because I had had such good results from following Dr. Clark's herbal recommendations after reading her first book, I was willing to step out of my comfort zone once again. This time I could barely comprehend the far-out research and experiments that Dr. Clark engaged in. But I had long since decided that, unless something was dangerous, I would be a willing guinea pig.

Dr. Clark explained her disovery in *The Cure for All Diseases*. "What makes me think I can find things in the human body that a blood test cannot? What new technology makes this possible? Why is electronic testing superior in many ways to chemical methods? What are my claims of electrically killing parasites based on?"

Dr. Clark never intended to profit or sell any of her discoveries. She was a true scientific researcher who hoped to help mankind. She stated she did not officially endorse any particular brand of "zapper." She detailed instructions in her book on how to build a zapper. Obviously very few people could construct one even with her detailed drawings.

I found a company called Healthy Signs which reported that they offered zappers used by Dr. Clark in her clinic designed and built to the specifications personally directed by Dr. Clark. I sent for mine, feeling quite silly and naïve. It arrived in a very small box.

Healthy Signs supplied literature along with the zapper. "Zapper" is the generic term for an electronic device invented by Dr. Hulda Clark, Ph.D., N.D. and her son Geoffrey in 1994.

"Utilizing a small harmless nine-volt battery, it emits a specific frequency that rids your body of parasites, bacteria, and viruses. But it takes more than one treatment. It takes three treatments to kill everything. Why? The first zapping kills viruses, bacteria, and parasites. But a few minutes later, bacteria and viruses (different ones) often recur. I concluded they had been infecting the parasites, and killing the parasites released them. The second zapping kills the released viruses and bacteria, but soon a few viruses appear again. They must have been infecting some of the last bacteria. After a third zapping, I never find any viruses, bacteria or parasites, even hours later."

I started to use the zapper, but I have to admit that I wasn't completely convinced this was legit, so I did not actually use it as directed. I wish I had because later in my struggle I turned to it with good results.

At this point I was improving albeit slowly, so I was open to trying new things, all the while doing as much research as possible. I was by now becoming convinced I had somehow contracted a microscopic parasitic organism, etiology unknown, that was raising havoc with my immune system. I was determined to make life miserable for these uninvited organisms. I would continue to search to find ways to starve them out of existence.

Thank you, God! I finally felt I turned the corner of a bad book. Could it be possible that help was available from God's Garden all along? I just had to find it.

Chapter Nine

The Power of Silver

FTER READING ABOUT THE HEALTH benefits of silver, I had become intrigued by the possible benefits of using this ancient and powerful natural antibiotic, antiseptic, and antibacterial liquid.

At Ancker Hospital—now Regions—as a student nurse, I remember putting silver nitrate in new-born babies' eyes to prevent blindness due to venereal disease.

Eye infections used to be a major cause of blindness in children, and were often caused by the same bacteria that caused gonorrhea or chlamydia in women. As a baby traveled through the birth canal, s/he could pick up bacteria present in the mother's vaginal secretions or fluids.

I also remember silver nitrate was being used in Ancker's burn unit to treat very severely burned patients with some excellent results. My good friend Faith Nelson O'Neill, R.N. was one of the first nurses assigned to the burn unit. She often spoke of the success they had under the guidance of the director Dr. James La Fave, M.D.

According to author Jacqueline Nasseff Hilgert, who wrote *Metamorphosis: a History of the Regions Hospital Burn Center*, published in 2015 by the Regions Hospital Foundation, Dr.Lafave studied with Carl Moyer, M.D. at Washington University in St. Louis, Missouri, where Moyer was using silver nitrate as an anti-bacterial treatment for burns. The compound was the same basic component used in photographic film. When Dr. LaFave returned to Ancker Hospital in St. Paul from St.

Louis in 1963, he designated a "burn unit" that became the ninth specialized burn center in the nation.

In an article published in the *St. Paul Pioneer Press* in 1965, LaFave explained burn treatment to reporter Albert Eisele:

For about the first 48 hours, the patient is in shock phase as he loses tremendous amounts of body fluids through the burned area. If these fluids aren't replaced, he goes into shock and may die. Once through the shock phase, the patient becomes susceptible to infection or burn wound sepsis. The big advantage of the silver nitrate treatment is that it controls burn wound sepsis.

Faith Nelson O'Neill said, "Almost all burn patients died of infection. There wasn't any specific, real good treatment. You'd use different kinds of bandages and different kinds of solutions, but they (the patients) almost always got infected. When a body suffers a burn injury, it will use its resources to heal tissue. Consequently, patient outcomes remained poor even as new treatments were brought online."

In the *Annals of Burns and Fire Disasters*, Volume XIII m.4, December, 2000, the Local Burn Unit, St. Joseph Hospital, Lisbon, Portugal reported: "Effective, topical antimicrobial agents decrease infection and mortality in burn patients. Silver sulphadiazine continues to be the antimicrobial agent most often used in burn facilities. Combined topical use of silver sulphadiazine and other antimicrobials may be a possible solution to bacterial resistance in burn wounds."

Mark Stengler, M.D. in his book, *The Natural Physician's Healing Therapies*, writes that he uses colloidal silver for the internal and external treatment of acute infections. He also uses it as an antifungal and antiparasitic agent, giving it to patients internally for infections of the digestive tract. "Other holistic doctors," he says, "use colloidal silver for the long-term treatment of Lyme Disease."

I wanted to try it, so I researched a company selling Colloidal Silver Generators advertised to make your own, safe, pure, therapeutic-quality colloidal silver solution whenever you need it. At the time I wanted to try it, natural health stores did not carry it. They do now however.

As soon as I received the generator, I started to administer the colloidal silver to myself according to data supplied by users' own accounts of what they were using. I felt this product arrested my symptoms more than anything else I had tried. Because I had been so sick, however, it could only help me as part of a multi-pronged approach. It turned out I needed a combination of herbs, antioxidants, vitamins, and cleansing products in addition to the colloidal silver to build up my body after the source of the infection was alleviated.

Chapter Ten

Ageless Remedies

MY SEARCH FOR A TOTAL CURE led me back into my local health food store, and I again talked to Joanie. I told her of my quest to return to good health, but I also admitted I was not there yet. She remembered a place in Colorado she might have information on. Luckily she did. It was Hanna's Herb Shop—Hanna Kroeger with her phone number.

My lucky day!

I called and Hanna actually answered. I told her my sad story, and she simply said I should send a sputum sample to her. As a registered nurse, I found all this contrary to my nursing background. But as a suffering, pitiful, helpless person, this was the path I must take. I complied. The results came in with a short shopping list. I ordered the items and started taking them as per Hanna's suggestions. They were homeopathics and vibropathics:

Literature included with my order stated, "Homeopathy has been used for nearly two hundred years all over the world. A great amount of search and documented clinical cases have shown that Homeopathy is exceptionally safe, effective and useful for most everyone. It is a naturopathic form of medicine, meaning it works with the body's own systems, energies and natural way of operating and functioning. Homeopathy does not override or divert the body; instead it assists the body's own healing energies."

Vibropathics: All are times six x potency.

I ordered these items from Hannas Herb Shop:

1. Epstein Barr-BE—Sound components to natural defense maintenance.

2. Protozoa—A large classification of single- celled organisms; protozoa are common in many environments.

3. Pancreatic Flukes—Basic food preparation and good hygiene help keep unwanted visitors away

4. Thyroid metabolizer—Maintain a balanced thyroid and metabolism. Works best along with lifestyle modifications, such as the elimination of caffeine, sugar, stress and poor nutrition.

5. Staph—Nutrition, exercise, rest and common sense are sound components to natural defense maintenance. Limited exposure to unfavorable conditions is also beneficial.

I felt better and better most of the time as I used these products. I knew what I was doing was working. But the damage must have been extensive because I continued to get flare-ups of previous symptoms at unpredictable intervals. These flare-ups were sometimes as painful as when my illness first began. I especially noticed the drilling pain in the back of my head and around my torso. I wasn't out of the woods yet. Also my eyes continued to give me a lot of trouble—the matting, difficulty seeing, blurriness, feeling as if sand was constantly in my eyes.

I was intrigued by this woman Hanna Kroeger who co-founded with her husband Rudolf Kroeger Hanna's Herb Shop in Boulder, Colorado. I had many telephone conversations with this remarkable woman, who was so unassuming and soft spoken and kind. She introduced me to the world of herbs and homeopathy. At the time I put my health in her hands, I was ready to try whatever she suggested. The black hole I was in was simply not acceptable. I trusted that someone somewhere must be able to tell me what to do. I thank God for directing me to Hanna.

She suggested some additional supplements and special teas. I also did a cleansing fast. The three-day fast consisted of:

*Eat pineapple and watermelon daily.
*Drink eight eight ounce glasses of steam-distilled water per day.
*Drink one cup of warm water to one squeezed lemon per day.
*Drink pure cranberry juice.
*Eat fresh apple sauce, mashed with a blender, not cooked.
*Take Spirulina, five tablets three times per day.

After the fast, I added these healing supplements, based on suggestions from Hanna Kroeger (*Traditional Herbals for Modern Living* by Hanna Kroeger).

1. Olive Leaf Extract. "Traditional folk literature credits it with a wide range of action to help fight infections."
2. Circu-Flow. "Helps maintain cardiovascular function and a healthy circulatory system."
3. Aloe Vera. "Laxative, intestinal difficulties, pain reliever, cell rejuvenator, burns, antiviral, immune system booster, general healing tonic."
4. Magnesium. "Magnesium is the fourth most abundant mineral in our bodies and is found primarily in our bones. This nutrient provides energy, regulates body temperature, helps you sleep, relaxes your muscles, and boosts your immune system."
5. Vitamin B6. (Pyridoxine) "Pyridoxine is involved in more bodily functions than almost any other single nutrient."

(The source of additional descriptives after numbered items is from *Prescription for Nutritional Healing*, by James F. Balch, M.D.)

As in every suggestion, Hanna carefully noted: "Bear in mind that the herbs listed are for prevention and maintenance and for problems that do not require major medical intervention. They are not intended to replace the expertise of a primary-care physician. If the complaint you are treating is not getting better, or if it is getting worse, consult a doctor."

I enjoyed reading Hanna's extensive booklets to get a glimpse of her voluminous, far reaching, innovative perception of God's gift to all of us that she saw so clearly. Rarely are true pioneers recognized for their efforts during their own time.

During the early years, Hanna made her own herb combinations at the kitchen table a few at a time. She gave her formulas away to anyone who needed help. She soon became known for her formulas and as a master of using subtle and unique combinations of two or more herbs to improve the whole system of the body. The herb combinations were to be a start she never imagined. In 1978 Hanna started Kroeger Herb products to keep up with the growing demand for her formulas. Over the years Kroeger Herb Products has grown beyond Hanna's original vision and nationally distributes Hanna's products.

I continued to receive Hanna's regular newsletter, *Herbal Insights*, and to this day I use her products. The Kroeger label is in many health food stores throughout the country.

I was never able to meet this dynamic health pioneer using natural healing methods but read of her life's work. It is astounding what she has contributed to the health and healing of thousands and thousands of suffering individuals.

Until her middle eighties, she wrote books, lectured, taught, formulated new products, helped people with their health problems, answered stacks of mail, conducted church services on Sundays, researched health and medical information, and answered phone calls all the while taking care of her family. Also, in her own words, she shared the workings of her inquisitive mind in her newsletter *Herbal Insights*.

In Summer 1998 issue, she wrote:

Dear Reader:
Though I've been holding the summertime retreat for more than 30 years, the work that went into getting started this May was exhausting. My people caution me to slow down, but that's really not my way. Even though there was paperwork and preparations, I didn't hesitate to run (maybe, "waddle quickly" is a better description) for the phone whenever it rang. I kept answering letters and kept church activities going, too.

How do I do it? God's energy that He supplies is limitless. You just have to get up early enough in the morning to find it. I still wake at 4:00 a.m. to honor Him. Though I don't have my husband Rudolph with me anymore, I connect with my beloved during Morning Prayer. Also, I have my sister, Beatrix, nearby. She's 92 and she's hoeing the garden right now! I also have my wonderful son and grandchildren helping every day. I'm fortunate to have loved ones and good work to do.

Here's another secret. You see the dandelions popping in your yard like little rascals? They're not the scourge you think. Rather than spraying them with harmful agents or chopping them up with the mower, recognize them as a symbol of spring's "wood energy." Also, look at my article inside to find the detoxifying properties of dandelion. Get ready to do some "spring cleaning" and stay young!

One last note, look in your mailboxes in July for a sample of my new monthly newsletter. It's a response to customer's requests for more information about health concerns.

Sadly this was Hanna's last newsletter . . . a postscript on the front page said: "To our customers: On May 7, 1998, Hanna Kroeger made her final embrace in this world, in peace in her 85th year, Hanna's boundless energy continued to drive her life's work as a healer and as a dedicated mentor who helps others. She maintained an exuberating pace of corresponding, writing, and teaching."

May she rest in peace.

Chapter Eleven

Similia Similibus
Center Homeopathy

BECAUSE HANNA COMBINED SO MANY different mediums for treating illnesses, homeopathy being one of them, and I had not been familiar with homeopathy, I attended a nurses conference held at St. Thomas College in St. Paul, Minnesota. It was sponsored by the National Center for Homeopathy. My sister Sue and her friend, both nurse practitioners, attended with me.

More than a year had passed since I contracted the undiagnosed disease. It was time to go back to school. In this instance just for a day.

The University of St. Thomas in St. Paul, Minnesota, was the location for Homeopathy: A Complementary Therapy. The instructor was Lia Bello R.N., F.N.P., who had twenty-two years' experience in homeopathic study, practice, and teaching. She was the founder and leader of the Homeopathic Nurses Association and was certified in Classical Homeopathy. She taught health professionals and consumers around the country.

The case statement that I received that day said, "Homeopathy is a safe, cost-effective form of medicine for a variety of health conditions throughout the continuum of care from pregnancy to the end of life without regard to age, gender, or occupation. Based on the Law of Similars as formalized by Samuel Hahnemann (1755 to 1843), a German physician, homeopathy uses extremely dilute doses of substances that have been found empirically to stimulate and support the body in its resolution of disease symptoms."

The day was spent acquainting us attendees with a foreign (at least to us) wellness system. There were segments on first aid, common

83

ailments, cell salts, Bach flower remedies, how to find the current remedy, understanding homeopathy for chronic disease, and references available for further study using the materials provided. I ordered the Nurses Standard Homeopathic Household kit by Hyland that I continue to use to this day. My grandchildren from baby on enjoyed dissolving the tiny tables under their tongues to alleviate many of their childhood illnesses and conditions.

Case in point—a neighbor jogging by our home very early one morning was frantically swatting a swarm of bees away from her. I was checking my paper box, and she ran up to me, asking for help. She said she had been stung three to four times on the back of her neck. She said she was very allergic to bee stings, and her epipen was at home. She could not get hold of her husband on her cellphone. She was so upset she could hardly dial his number.

I ran into my home and grabbed my calming healing oils and she rubbed the lotion on her neck. I then asked her if she would like to try the two homeopathic remedies for bee stings from my nurse's kit. She said yes and took them according to the label directions. Her husband shortly arrived with her epipen (epinephrine injections to use for a life-threatening allergic reaction). If the epipen had not been available, these homeopathic remedies could have given her more time to get to an emergency room or possibly even take care of the emergency.

Most recently when flying I was seated in an aisle seat. A very large man sat next to me, squeezing his large frame into the tiny middle seat and holding his arms tight so not to offend his two seatmates. We exchanged hellos and settled in for the three-hour-plus flight. About an hour into the flight, this man suddenly became symptomatic of what appeared to be a terrible cold. Lots of blowing and coughing and distress. My seat mate and I tried to ignore his plight, not wanting to embarrass him.

After two-plus hours into the flight, I reached into my purse and checked if I had packed any remedies. I only had two—Bach Original Flower Essences CERATO for naturally occurring nervous tension and my homemade healing oils consisting of Arnica, almond oil, aloe vera jelly with a few drops of five different Aromatherapy Pure Essential Oils I used for calming and relaxation.

I asked the distressed man if he was getting a cold. No, he said. Do you have allergies? No, he said. "What do you think is happening to you?" He said he didn't know, but he flew a lot and this had never happened before. I explained what I had in my purse and would he like to try it. He said yes. I added several drops of the CERATO to his coke and put the oils into his hand and instructed him to rub it on his neck. I really wasn't sure if any of this would help him. But in ten minutes, I realized that his fits of coughing and blowing had subsided. I asked him if he was better, and he said yes, looking unsure what all had happened. The last hour of the flight he was quiet, and we who were seatmates surrounding him were very relieved as well.

Over the years I have repeated a similar scenario with family and friends in response to different emergencies or conditions. I have experienced many "every day miracles" that occurred regularly with homeopathic remedies—the sprained ankle that healed in record time and the patient who shows very little bruising after a major surgery after using arnica, the flu remedy that shortened a person's misery, a sleep remedy that helped even chronic insomnia, an allergy formula that relieves sniffing, and many others. Doctors especially in Europe are quite fond of using these remedies in their practices because they sometimes work very well.

Although the practice of medicine is regulated under law, the use of homeopathic medicines for self-care of acute ailments is available to all, and those who keep a homeopathic kit in their house for domestic emergencies, are free, under the laws of most states, to use them in such situations.

Because of the research necessary to write this chapter of my book I found to my astonishment that my instructor at the nurses' seminar I took in 1997, Lia Bello, F.N.P., and C.C.H., continues her practice in Santé Fe, New Mexico. Lia is the founder of the Homeopathic Nurse

Association and is America's foremost homeopathic nurse educator. Lia has taught the same course hundreds of times over the forty years since she first learned homeopathy and is glad to share it with others. Lia loves to open up the world of homeopathy to mothers, nurses, and other health-care practitioners. Residing in Sante Fe, New Mexico, Lia has a private practice specializing in holistic health care.

I wrote this note to her.

Dear Lia.

In 1997 you instructed a class at St. Thomas College in St. Paul, Minnesota entitled: Homeopathy: Complementary Therapy. I attended. (I am a trained R.N.) I kept your class notes all these years.

Now I am writing a medical memoir entitled *No Diagnosis*.

I would like your permission to include some of your materials that were provided at your seminar.

When searching for your current address I was pleased to see you are still very active with the Homeopathic community.

During my illness and subsequent recovery, I used Homeopathy along with other complementary therapies.

Thank you very much for your consideration of my request.

Shortly after I received Lia's reply via email.
November 13, 2015
Subject: Homeopathy
Hi Karen, please do visit my website and read articles, etc. Here is the Emotion Code Book—I clear people's trapped emotions—if they have them—while also treating them with their constitutional remedy.

Lia also graciously responded to my request to include some of her data in my chapter. She has given me permission to use anything from her web site in this chapter on Similia Similbus.

I have selected points of interest from her web site in order to give a synopsis of the elementary points she covers. "Homeopathy is a system of natural medicine used by millions of people worldwide for more than 200 years to achieve wellness."

Evidence Based Homeopathy. "A health technology assessment report on homeopathy commissioned by the Swiss government, has concluded that homeopathy is clinically effective, cost-effective and safe. This H.T.A report exhaustively reviews the scientific literature and its unambiguous, positive conclusions have resulted in homeopathy being included on the list of medical treatments which are reimbursed through Switzerlands national health insurance. It summarizes twenty two reviews, twenty of which show positive results for homeopathy."

As the use of Homeopathy increases in their positive results as well, the medical establishment will be forced to eventually acknowledge the contributions to wellness this field makes.

PART II

A Cure without a Diagnosis

Chapter Twelve

Wrap Up: Almost Well, But Detours Ahead

T HIS PERIOD WAS A PIECE OF CAKE compared to the initial onset of this disease and the fits and starts of my route to recovery. I had a plan at least and a course of action and treatments available to me. I was no longer confused and desperate. I no longer needed to present myself as a needy patient to anyone, and I calmly accepted my condition and knew that I had a diagnosis even though it was self-applied at this point.

My journaling continued even though as throughout my illness none of my symptoms made sense.

As an example, on September 18th, 1997, I made this entry: "I developed black and blue spots. They were the size of a small orange on the back of my calves and also the back of my thighs. I developed a positive Homans sign (when the leg is outstretched and you bring up your toes you feel pain). I also had almost constant pain in my chest and left knee. My nurse daughter, Deborah, became very concerned when I told her of my symptoms this morning. She said it could be a warning of early deep vein thrombosis (*D.V.T.*) of the lower leg.

"Ultra Sound ordered due to symptoms. It was non-conclusive. I very much appreciated my daughter's concern about me and following through by calling my doctor. In my altered state, I didn't even grasp the potential seriousness of *D.V.T.* since I was having one strange symptom after another. Besides what's another one anyway?

"Continuing on anti-parasitic program of wormwood, black walnut, cloves, and ornithine."

On November 1st, I experienced a happy day with this entry: "So much better!!!! My eyes are even better, but some exudate still present. Stools finally normal. Some itching yet, especially the back of my head. But THANK YOU, GOD! I CAN LIVE WITH THIS! I feel I was saved by God's own Garden and his angels that walk among us. I now had great empathy for other hurting and sick people."

On November 20th, 1997: "To stay on Synthroid for now and recheck in three months."

On February 23rd, 1998: "Appointment to see Dr. H., eye doctor at the University of Minnesota. He noted that my plugs were gone. They probably dissolved. They can slip into nasal cavities and even come out through the nose. I still experienced lots of tearing from my left eye, and Dr. H. noticed I had unusual dryness in my right eye. He said my eyes were better but sorry to say my vision wasn't. Since July 1996 my vision had become much worse for reading, and now I always needed glasses to read while before the onset of my illness I did not.

On June 15th, 1998, I wrote: "Happily I can report that I am lots lots better, but some symptoms remain: Black and blue spots (large) that got ugly and yellow and were sore to the touch, profuse bleeding in my mouth (lip) that was hard to stop. I put Echinacea on a wet towel and held it tight to stop the bleeding, and still some discharge from my eyes."

In October of 1998, I wrote: "Because I wanted a fresh start with a medical doctor who would not be privy to my unusual disease, I transferred to a different clinic. I took all my medical records from my previous clinic but did not transfer them to my new clinic. I was almost well now and wanted my new doctor to see the present instead of the awful past I had just gone through. I told my new doctor that I had a bad experience with an undiagnosed auto-immune type disease and wanted a fresh start. My new doctor has been wonderful, and it feels good to not have to go over any of that nightmare illness. I am now a well person with the exception of a few diagnoses:
- Hypothyroidism.
- Fuchs dystrophy (eye disease) and dry eye."

On May 22, 1999, I wrote: "Two years since the sudden death of my dear father, we have added a joyful event. Our son Jeff married his beautiful bride, Kari. It was a spectacular wedding and reception and a grand celebration with three of our four parents able to attend."

In December of that year, I wrote: "Joyful entry as we are now happy grandparents of another beautiful baby—our little Brooke was born to our son Dan and his wife, Linda. She is a marvelous, exquisite baby with dark, curly hair. I took care of her big sister, Paige, while Brooke was born and took her to see her new little sister. We are so grateful for the miracle of her birth.

The spring of 2000 to present: "We sold our business and experienced a flurry of adjusting to retirement with realigning and readjusting in our lives. We also were blessed with six more delightful grandchildren. Praise the Lord!

Lauren was born October 2000, Blake born January 2003, Gracie born February 2004, Lucia born May 2004, Henri born January 2007, and Luke born February 2008. With the birth of our each grandbaby, I gratefully celebrated my privilege of being able to give each grandchild my grandma's blessing with the sign of the cross on their tiny foreheads. We have been busy being proud grandparents and have tried to spend as much time with all of them as possible. I also was feeling much better, so this time I could hug and squeeze them without worry about them catching something.

"The Lords unfailing love and mercy still continues fresh as the morning, as sure as the sunrise." Lamentations 3:22-23 Good News Bible

By the fall of 2000, I could write: "Almost a year has gone by with no entries in my health journal!

"Obviously I am a lot better. I even gained all my weight back and more and had to diet to get rid of five pounds. I have developed a very guarded approach to the medical establishment, however, and distrust the heavy influence of the pharmaceutical industry in doctor's medical practices. Sad to think of all their patients with similar symptoms will *never* be helped with their methods. I want to help as many sick people as possible find a way back to health but will need to research and learn more before I can give too much advice. All I know is that I am back to health (almost) and owe it mostly to Alternative Medicine. 'Almost' means I continue to have eye (dark) matting (especially my right eye). It's closed up when I wake up during the night and in the morning. I still have a few sharp twinges deep within the back of my head. I realize it will take constant diligence to get my health back totally. Once or twice a year I continue to cleanse as maintenance with wormwood, black walnut, and cloves. I now use a purchased kit available at many health food stores and even some grocery stores that have health food sections. It is called Paragon by Renew Life. I add additional cloves and Pau de 'Arco, a probiotic, and a fiber supplement.

"When I get bronchitis or sinus symptoms, I use a nasal spray bottle and add colloidal silver with a drop of eucalyptus and squirt it deep into each nostril each morning and evening. I also take colloidal silver when I start to get sick with anything. I take an assortment of anti-oxidants and herbal supplements.

"But I now have my life back with the realization that I most likely will always have this auto-immune condition that may lead to diseases, which, hopefully, I can manage.

"My beautiful mother, Veronica, died on April 25th, 2011, at age ninety-one. All five of us children were at her bedside. I also did her eulogy as a gift to her. She continues to send roses to us as her favorite red rose bush blooms prolifically from early spring until mid-October here in Minnesota.

"My beautiful mother-in-law, Rose, died on May 9th, 2013, at the age of 100. Her granddaughter Sue did her eulogy. She was a treasure.

"My amazing father-in-law, Tony, died at the age of 103 on October 25th, 2014. He was our patriarch. Bob did his father's eulogy and did him proud.

"They are greatly missed as well as my Father Joe.

"I do now have a few diagnosed illnesses to live with: Hypothyroidism, for which I take medication and see an excellent general practitioner; Fuchs Dystrophy (eye disease) and cateracts (mild) both eyes, for which I take anti-allergy ophthalmic drops twice daily and have yearly visits with my eye doctor. If symptoms accelerate I may be a candidate for a corneal transplant, but for now just maintenance; Cataracts (mild) in both eyes. I see an excellent eye specialist; Atrial fibrillation (A-fib), for which I take medication, including a 81-mg aspirin and see an excellent cardiologist; and Polymyalgia and giant cell arteritis, for which I take medication and see an excellent rheumatologist.

"Note: Infrequently I have had attacks of atrial fibrillation and have some fast-acting medication I can take to stop the symptoms. Several times I needed to go to the emergency room and was hospitalized twice for stabilization. As I have aged and added diseases, I have followed accepted protocol and am being seen by specialists.

"Most recently I was given a diagnosis of early-stage breast cancer that will set me off on another journey that so many of my friends and some family members have already been on. This illness comes with a diagnosis and a well-researched plan of treatment with superb doctors I am confident will give me the words 'cancer free.' I will supplement prescribed medications with integrative, alternative and functional medicine as per my doctors okay.

"All in all, my health has become a side issue to living, a happy result, which is wonderful. During the middle of my fight for my life, it became my every waking thought."

"We know that in all things God works for good with those who love Him, those for whom he has called according to His purpose."
Romans 8:28 Good News Bible

Lord, I can face the future with confidence, knowing that all the events of all my tomorrows are in your loving hands. For this hope, I thank you.

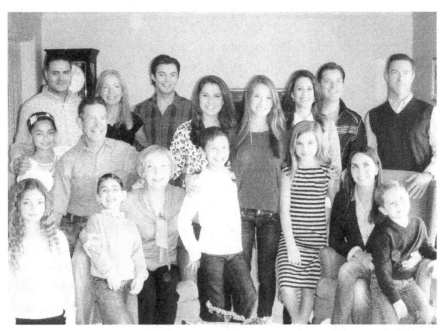

Ament Family, Thanksgiving, 2013

PART III

Unraveling the Mystery

Chapter Thirteen

Merging Conventional, Integrative, Alternative and Functional Medicine

I NTEGRATIVE MEDICINE IS alternative medicine used together with conventional medicine treatment in a belief (not by the use of a scientific method) that it complements (improves the results of the treatment).

Obviously conventional medicine has given us a quality of medical care unsurpassed in the modern world. The inroads into bio-medical and cutting-edge surgical techniques has been phenomenal. We are beneficiaries of the largesse available to us. But in some respects, the division of medicine into defined specialties has eliminated the ability of our physicians to see the whole person. Without the whole-person approach, the practice of medicine sometimes labels a patient according to the textbook definition, and, at that point, the patient starts on a path of incorrect if not downright harmful treatments. A case in point is the diagnosis of psychosis based on a simple statement of bug bites, not taking into account a whole slew of systemic symptoms and past history of totally non-eventful medical complaints. This can even have us go back to the dark ages where diagnosis and treatment is concerned.

Dr. Andrew Weil, M.D., author of *Spontaneous Healing* is one of the world's leading proponents of integrative medicine. In his book he says, "Using synthetic drugs and surgery to treat health conditions was known just a few decades ago as simply, 'medicine.' Today, this system is increasingly being termed 'conventional medicine.' This is the kind of medicine most Americans still encounter in hospitals and clinics. Any therapy that is typically excluded by conventional medicine, and that patients use instead of conventional medicine, is known as 'alternative medicine.' An alternative medicine practice that is used in conjunction with a conventional one is known as 'complementary' medicine. Together, complementary and alternative medicines are often referred to by the acronym CAM. As defined by the National Center for complementary and alternative medicine at the National Institutes of Health, integrative medicine 'combines mainstream medical therapies and CAM therapies for which there is some high-quality scientific evidence and effectiveness.'"

A family friend of ours, Dr. Mark Hallstrom, M.D., is in practice at the Integracare/Williams Clinics in Sartell, Minnesota. He is a bright young physician who is able to offer his patients an approach to improving patient outcomes across a wide range of chronic health conditions through careful analysis of common underlying pathways that interact to produce disease and dysfunction of health and vitality.

I called Mark to discuss the writing of this book, No Diagnosis, and briefly explained the reasons I was writing it. He graciously presented me with a copy of his personal book, *Just Be Well* by Thomas A. Sult, M.D., and a loan of one of his medical textbooks, which I perused carefully and returned. I loved the book and enjoyed the interesting one on one integrative approach that Dr. Sult used with his patients.

Dr. David S. Jones, M.D., president of the Institute for Functional Medicine wrote the foreword and captured the essence of Sult's book perfectly.

"In *Just Be Well*, Dr. Sult illustrates what functional medicine, a systems medicine approach to chronic illnesses can mean and do for patients in the exam room of clinical medicine. Using and understanding the fundamental organizational and physiological processes within each of us as key nodes of biological influence allows doctors to find the underlying causes of disease. When properly in balance, these processes yield wellness; when out of balance, our body's system devolves into dysfunction and disease. Through a robust and disciplined process of inquiry, we can discover the underlying causes of patient's illnesses."

In a nutshell, *Just Be Well*, by Thomas A. Sult, M.D. is a book for seekers of vibrant health.

The future holds hope for an expansion of the myriad of health systems that are finding acceptance among the general public due to RE-SULTS. Young people today are paying attention to what works and what does not for them. They are much more open than the traditionalists that have gone before them to exploring other modalities.

Years ago it would have been unthinkable to graduate from a four-year college and then to apply for admission to Bastyr University in Seattle, Washington, to complete a degree in Naturopathic Medicine and Traditional Chinese Medicine. But a young couple from St. Cloud, Minnesota, have plans to do just that. They are Jordan and Ariel K. Jordan will be pursuing Naturopathic medicine and Ariel Traditional Chinese Medicine at Bastyr University. They are excited to be able to work towards, not just careers, but a means to heal and care for the whole person and be able to practice preventative medicine.

Bastyr.edu offers a range of graduate, undergraduate and certificate programs in ten distinct areas of study. Areas of study include naturopathic medicine, acupuncture, Oriental medicine, nutrition, ayurveda sciences, midwifery, counseling and psychology, exercise, science, holistic landscaper design, and herbal sciences.

They and others like them are the future of wellness medical care using CAM (Complementary, Alternative Medicine).

Amazing changes have developed in the world of medicine since I became ill in 1996. Many traditional modalities have evolved and strengthened to the benefit of the patients. State of the art facilities are now available in many communities to treat cancer, heart, bone, and other specialties. Our community is very fortunate to have access to these networks.

But as much as things have changed for the better, people that experience symptoms similar to mine in 1996 still have nowhere to go. They are still falling between the cracks in the medical field, and, most alarming, some are still diagnosed as having a psychotic disorder if they make the mistake of telling their doctors the unusual, bizarre symptoms they are having. Twenty-one years of cries for help and still stuck in limbo.

"Let food be thy medicine and medicine be thy food."

Hippocrates

"If people let the government decide what foods they eat and what medicines they take, their bodies will soon be in as sorry a state as the souls who live under tyranny."

Thomas Jefferson

Chapter Fourteen

Cries for Help
Across the Pond

As darkness falls upon me,
I feel the dreaded feeling that
Encompasses my whole being
And fills me with emptiness

Those feelings rush in . . .
The ones that leave me exhausted
From trying to fight and win
A battle that is raging in my entire body.

Cries for help go unheard.
The pain far outweighs anything
That anyone can ever relate to.
Very few know this kind of pain.

As hard as the physical pain is,
The other pain is so much deeper.
It stems from a rejection that others can't fathom.
It is unbearable but somehow makes me stronger.

It is becoming increasingly difficult
To hide the demon that has taken over.
Trying to act normal is a struggle and only
Makes others question my conveyed helplessness.

Being alone is comforting
I can cry and nobody will pity me.
I have become my own best friend
And I love and hate myself concurrently.

Judgment comes from all sides
And has taken so much from my soul,
I haven't the strength to fight much longer.
Yet the only answer is not an option.

Sleep is so difficult
The unconscious mind is as full of pain
As my body and nothing will mask it.
Please. I must rest and sleep in order to fight.

As the darkness fades to light
I am once again facing another battle.
Sunshine helps to focus but fighting alone
Has still left me in the daytime dark.

My thoughts are jumbled, my head a fog . . .
It keeps me from being who I am.
Many do not know the real me . . .
You possibly never will.

I see and feel and think things that I hate
My brain is full of garbage.
What once was functioning brilliantly
Is now filled with mindless trails of sorrow.

The days are short and empty
With few bright spots to sustain me.
As the sun lowers in the west, I find myself
Once again facing the darkness that I despise.

And as the cycle begins again
The cycle of highs and lows,
Pain and more pain, the actions of a fool . . .
So much that I can't remember from day to day.

In this hour of this day, I ask you Lord for guidance
Through my unrelenting maze of confusion and anger.
May I have the strength to keep going, fighting, and
Struggling to make others understand.

Composed by Patricia in 2004. Patricia gave permission for all to read and share on the Morgellons UK Awareness Campaign 2010 web site http://www.morgellonsuk/symptoms.htm

Chapter Fifteen

Mary Leitao, Biologist, Researcher, Persistent Concerned Mother

Morgellons Research Foundation MRF

ANY OF YOU READERS WILL never have heard of Morgellons. Consider yourself very fortunate. For those of you who think you may have it or know someone who does, you can easily identify with Patricia.

In the throes of my own symptoms, I could have written every one of these pleading utterances to anyone and everyone, hoping against hope that someone would pick up the trail of symptoms equaling discovery and, viola, a cure for myself perhaps but certainly for many others afflicted. Patricia is a poet extraordinaire. I pray that she found a cure and peace of mind and body.

Sadly her words written in 2004 are still applicable now.

I will try to track the time line of discovery and attempts by sufferers to help each other, hoping against hope that the CDC or Mayo clinic or a researcher would break through this wall of impossibility and give these people a diagnosis other than a catch all phrase "delusional parasitosis."

Much is said about the progress of science in these centuries. I should say that the useful results of science have accumulated, but there has been no accumulation of knowledge, strictly speaking, for posterity . . . for knowledge to be acquired only by corresponding experience. How can we know what we are told merely? Each man can interpret another's experience only by his own.

"He is not a true man of science who does not bring some sympathy to his studies, and expect to learn something by behavior as well as application. The process of discovery is very simple. An unwearied and systematic application of known laws to nature causes the unknown to reveal themselves. Almost any mode of observation will be successful at last, for what is most wanted is method."
Henry David Thoreau

In 2002 six years after I developed Morgellons-like symptoms, Mary Leitao, mother of a two-year-old boy, noticed her son had sores on his lips and complained of "bugs." Mary was uniquely qualified to pursue this strange complaint. She had a Bachelor of Science degree in biology and was a former lab technician. Her husband, Edward, was an internist at a hospital in Pittsburg.

She amassed a pile of medical records while consulting with many physicians, trying to determine what could possibly be happening to her son. No one believed her. An infectious disease specialist at Johns Hopkins University suggested it was a case of Munchausen's by proxy, a psychiatric syndrome in which a parent pretends her child is sick to get attention from the medical system.

As any concerned mother would do, she was not content to let her son suffer without getting him help and relief. In 2004 after hours and hours of studiously trying to connect the dots, her research led her to a seventeenth-century French medical article describing an illness called Morgellons that exhibited symptoms similar to her sons.

Mary had now provided the link between this ancient disease and her own son's illness and assumed the ancient name of Morgellons for this twenty-first century malady.

After putting up a website describing her son's illness, she was surprised to find that thousands of people responded with like symptoms. They poured out their stories and their frustrations and nonbelief of the ridiculous symptoms they were having. And they particularly shared their sadness that their doctors had absolutely no idea what to do for them.

One would think this discovery would have hastened the discovery and subsequent relief for thousands of like sufferers but this was not to be. She had hit a wall of refusal by the medical community to give credence to her discovery, and, in fact, they were not very interested and sometimes downright hostile to the sufferers. They preferred to call this condition a psychiatric disorder and labeled it delusional parasitosis. Ultimately they wanted to treat these patients with psychiatric drugs.

This has created tremendous conflict between sufferers and their doctors that sadly continues to this day.

Mary started the Morgellons Research Foundation (MRF) in 2002 (informally) and as an official non-profit in 2004. The MRF stated on its website that its purpose was to raise awareness and funding for research into the proposed condition, described by the organization as a "poorly understood illness, which can be disfiguring and disabling."

She stated that she initially hoped to receive information from scientists or physicians who might understand the problem, but, instead, thousands of others contacted her describing their sores and fibers, as well as neurological symptoms, fatigue, muscle and joint pain, and other symptoms. The MRF is said to have received self-identified reports of Morgellons from all fifty states and fifteen other countries, including Canada, the U.K., Australia, and the Netherlands, and states that it has been contacted by over twelve thousand families.

In 2012 the Morgellons Research Foundation closed down and directed future inquires to Oklahoma State University, Dr. Randy Wymore. Dr. Wymore's research continues at OCU-CHS.

Chapter Sixteen

Media Coverage

NEWS SOURCE JENNA LEE on Fox TV on January 25, 2012, did a special on the mysterious disease with fibers and "things" crawling on them . . . real or in their heads? Dr. Manny Alveraz weighed in. It was reported that the CDC's study cost $600,000.00 . . . still a very small sum for a possible worldwide epidemic. It also was reported that the CDC looked at 109 patients, which is a paltry number considering that up to 20,000 people have registered with the CDC with Morgellon-like symptoms.

I was upset that the subject seemed to be lightly dismissed, and Dr. Alveraz focused on anxiety, mood disorders, and the power of the mind that can make you physically ill, mass hysteria? Nothing infectious.

I felt that Fox News told only a small part of the story and needed to hear "the rest of the story." So, I wrote to them:

Fox News
1211 Avenue of the Americas
New York, 0036-8795
Jenna Lee
Subject Morgellons

Dear Jenna,
Greetings to you!
Fox News is always on at our home and yesterday (January 26th) I heard a teaser ad at 10:00 a.m. that indicated there would be a special coming up soon on "people experiencing a mysterious disease with fibers and things crawling on them . . . real or in their heads?"

You then shuddered with the very thought seeming surreal and unimaginable.

I was glued to the television until 11:00 a.m. (Central Time) when Dr. Manny Alveraz came on as your guest. I had always enjoyed his past visits and loved his humor and clear thinking but the opinions he expressed yesterday made me exasperated and dismayed.

Physicians take a Hippocratic Oath to first do no harm to their patients. To the thousands and thousands of "Morgellons" sufferers, including young children, he did immeasurable harm to the hope that the medical community would soon offer them a cure. He instead repeated what many of their doctors had often told them that "the power of the mind can make you physically ill."

A little research on real "Morgellons sufferers" would quickly show that many if not most of these cases came on quickly and usually the previously "normal person" would actually remember the exact date and time that their life changed to a nightmare.

I should know. I am in the process of writing a medical memoir of a five-year odyssey of strange baffling beginnings of a mysterious disease that led to a multitude of systemic symptoms that were at times bizarre and sadly unrecognized by many if not most of the medical experts I consulted who, in much if not most of the time, labeled me as a person with a causative illness as perhaps, "making this up." This saga led me to search and assemble and use totally previously foreign Naturopathic remedies (I'm a former R.N.) with amazing results and a cure!

I am now healed with God's great help and feel the need to share and even help many people still struggling with similar symptoms and perhaps light a fire under some medical professionals to focus on my unusual case and draw parallels to a patient or patients of their own. The CDC (Center for Disease Control) is now studying up to 20,000 registrants with similar symptoms with, so far, no published results and no diagnoses and no apparent cures. (Note: Dr. Manny noted that the CDC actually spent $600,000.00 on the study of only 109 patients.) Considering how widespread this disease is and the ramifications of this spreading throughout the general public this is actually a pittance.

Mass hysteria? The power of the mind can do wonders, but, Doctor, many of these people have physical symptoms! They are all strangely similar to other sufferers thousands of miles away and until the day of infection they were leading normal lives.

Jenna, please follow through with the REST OF THE STORY and interview Gregory V. Smith, M.D., FAAP, or Mary Leitao the

Morgellons Research Foundations's director (whose small son contracted it), or Randy S. Wymore, Oklahoma Center for the Investigation of Morgellons disease.

Many Morgellons sufferers are at the end of their tolerance to
manage this illness. And in many if not most of the cases, these poor
people do end up with systemic symptoms that can often times be
lethal! Then they finally get their long sought out "medical diagnosis."

Please give them a little hope that something is being done somewhere.

Thank you so much.
Sincerely,
Karen Ament

Authors' note: I did not hear back.

Chapter Seventeen

CDC Savior or

Superior Antagonist?

January, 25, 2012
USA. Gov
1600 Clifton Road
Atlanta, GA. 30329-4027

Centers for Disease Control and Prevention
CDC Study of an Unexplained Dermopathy published in the Public
Library of Science (PLoS) One. Public Domain
Clinical, epidemiologic, histopathologic and molecular features of
an unexplained dermopathy

"Unexplained medical conditions can cause serious illness and disability among individuals, as well as demands on health care resources. In January 2008, CDC began an investigation that sought to better understand an unexplained apparent dermopathy, commonly referred to as Morgellons. CDC partnered with Kaiser Permanente (KP) in Northern California, a large group health plan in an area where many possible cases had been reported, and the Armed Forces Institute of pathology, to begin a comprehensive clinical and laboratory study of this condition."

The investigators contacted patients among KP-Northern California enrollees who had reported symptoms that included abnormal skin sensations or sores along with the presence of fibers in the affected skin areas. Included among these patients were some who used the term Morgellons to describe their condition. The objective of the investigation was to identify any possible common cause or risk factors for the condition. Investigators also sought to objectively describe signs and symptoms of this condition, study biopsy specimens from patients' skin sores, and examine fibers or other materials reported by patients as being on or in their skin.

Results of the study, published in PLoS One, show this condition appears to be uncommon among a population representative of Northern California residents. Skin damage from the sun was the most common skin abnormally found, and no single underlying medical condition or infectious source was identified. Upon thorough analysis, most sores appeared to result from chronic scratching and picking, without an underlying cause. The materials and fibers obtained from skin-biopsy specimens were mostly cellulose, compatible with cotton fibers.

Nueropsychological testing revealed a substantial number of study participants who scored high in screening tests for one or more co-existing psychiatric or additive conditions, including depression, somatic concerns (an indicator of preoccupation with health issues), and drug use.

This comprehensive study of an unexplained apparent dermopathy demonstrated no infectious cause and no indication that it would be helpful to perform additional testing for infectious diseases as a potential cause.

Future efforts should focus on helping patients reduce their symptoms through careful attention to treatment of co-existing medical, including psychiatric conditions that might be contributing to their symptoms.

Rebuttal:

After a decade of pleadings and plausible accounts of very believable strangely similar accounts of an abrupt onset terrifying disease by thousands and thousands of people the CDC grudgingly put together a study very halfheartedly. They spent a paltry sum of less than $600,000 and only interviewed 115 people and only forty were given a battery of physical and psychological tests that stretched over several days. This left thousands patiently waiting on their mail-in list, including myself. Obviously there was no urgency to hurry up in any way and no concern for the possibility that this could be an emerging disease possibly epidemic in nature. Hello, does anyone care out there?

It's very hard to imagine how the release of the long awaited study showing delusional parasitosis can possibly be believed for very long. The lists of sufferer's keeps increasing and soon, hopefully very soon, the sheer numbers of sufferers will garner attention again and the

CDC will have to address the issue again this time in a credible manner and with real urgency and with egg on their faces and their credibility below the low water mark.

TIMELINE OF CDC FACT FINDING

2006 - CDC task force consisting of twelve people formed.

2006 June - First meeting due to volume of concern about the syndrome.

2007 August 1 - CDC issued statement.

2007 November - CDC announced investigation under way. (Website opened up . . . Unexplained Dermopathy).

2008 January 25 - Petition circulated to request the CDC to investigate (by the Morgellons Research Foundation).

2008 June 17 - CDC enlisted aid of US Armed Forces.

2008 June 21 - *Washington Times* article . . . CDC enlists military to study mysterious, frightening skin ailment by Jennifer Harper.

2009 November 4 - CDC issued preliminary report.

2011 March 24 - CDC completed data analysis.

2012 January 25 - CDC Released results of study to find no infectious or environmental links.

2012 January 26 - Future Tense/Torie Bosch Editor shared comments on the results of the study.

2012 February 2 - CDC/Kaiser "Groundbreaking "Morgellons study a fraud by Cliff Mickelson.

These time lines are not necessarily inclusive but are listed to show the amount of time it took for the CDC to reach their conclusions.

Additional data on the chronological series of events that transpired before, during and after the CDC study:

The Morgellons Research Foundation sponsored an Advocacy Media Page and included a Sample letter to the media regarding the CDC study.

"I am writing to ask you to help inform the public and health professionals about a newly emerging disease called Morgellons disease.

Thousands of people's lives have been affected by this serious and devastating disease, and I am asking you to please help raise awareness."

On August 1, 2007, the CDC issued the following statement: "Morgellons is an unexplained and debilitating condition that has emerged as a public health concern. Recently, the Centers for Disease Control and Prevention (CDC) has received an increased number of inquiries from the public, health care providers, public health officials, Congress, and the media regarding this condition. Persons who suffer from this condition report a range of coetaneous symptoms including crawling, biting and stinging sensations; granules, threads or black speck-like materials on or beneath the skin; and/or skin lesions (e.g., rashes or sores) and some sufferers also report systemic manifestations such as fatigue, mental confusion, short-term memory loss, joint pain, and changes in vision. Moreover, some who suffer from this condition appear to have substantial morbidity and social dysfunction, which can include decreased work productivity or job loss, total disability, familial estrangement, divorce, loss of child custody, home abandonment, and suicidal ideation." The CDC further calls this disease an "emerging public health problem."

It is difficult to understand the tremendous suffering caused by the disease. Many people report feeling abandoned by the medical community as they experience increasingly bizarre, disfiguring and painful symptoms, while often being unable to receive medical treatment for their condition. A large number of patients become financially devastated and without health insurance because they can no longer work. Most people who suffer from Morgellons disease report feeling frightened and helpless.

Please contact the Morgellons Research Foundation for more information."

Since I contracted my disease in 1996, thousands and thousands of others before and after must have done so as well. There must be numerous longtime suffering people in agony. Many of these people must have consulted with numerous medical doctors regarding their symptoms as I had. Wouldn't one think that the CDC would have become more active in investigating this potentially catastrophic illness that could potentially affect many, many people? But no, they were either totally unaware of the turmoil or ignored the sufferers because they had already placed them in the DOP box and why bother?

Their long awaited investigation and report appeared to be a method of quieting the opposition (i.e. sufferers and their advocates).

While reading the January 21, 2008, *Washington Times,* an article jumped out at me entitled, "CDC enlists military to study mysterious, frightening skin ailment" by Jennifer Harper. Finally the CDC was responding . . . thank heavens . . . soon there would be an answer to all this misery.

The Washington Times
"CDC enlists military to study mysterious, frightening skin ailment" By Jennifer Harper (with files from CDC historical archives press briefing transcripts. Released by Dave Daigle with CDC's press office on January 16th, 2008.)

The Centers for Disease Control and Prevention (CDC) officially calls it the "unexplained illness." On January 16th, 2008, the federal agency announced it would formally investigate the condition-known as Morgellons syndrome—and is bringing in the military to help it do it.

The cause and risk factors are unknown, though most of the cases are showing up in California, Florida and Texas, said Dr. Michele Pearson, CDC's principal investigator. The agency is spending $545,000 and enlisting the help of the U.S. Armed Forces Institute of Pathology as well as the American Academy of Dermatology to conduct "immediate" and "rigorous" research.

There is no textbook definition on this condition. There are many hypotheses about what might be causing and contributing to it. So it's a frustrating journey, not only for patients but for providers who care for them," Dr. Pearson said.

"Clearly, the suffering these patients are experiencing is real," he added.

Public awareness of the condition has been intensifying.

Morgellons was first identified in 2002 by Mary M. Leitao, a biologist whose toddler displayed the spectrum of disgusting symptoms. She established the New York- based Morgellons Research Foundation (MRF) after failing to find what she considered appropriate care for her 2 year- old son. The advocacy group has since registered more than 11,000 people who say they have the condition or have been mistreated by the medical community.

Some doctors have dismissed Morgellons as dermatitis, hives, scabies or "delusional parasitosis," in which patients are obsessed with the idea that their bodies have been invaded by parasites—prompting them to seek unconventional cures. Some desperate victims have swallowed veterinary deworming medicines or rubbed bleach on affected skin.

Limited research has revealed a potential between Morgellons and the same bacteria that causes Lyme disease, according to the American Journal of Clinical Dermatology. To date, treatments have included antipsychotic drugs, antibiotics, antifungals, herbal supplements and light therapy. Morgellons cases have appeared in Canada, Australia and several European countries, though the CDC has not established that the syndrome is common in "underdeveloped countries."

The MRF, meanwhile, has long urged self-identified victims to write to public officials and contact the press.

The strategy has worked. Global interest spiked in 2006 after a series of alarming prime-time reports appeared on CNN, NBC and particularly ABC – where Morgellons was showcased on "Medical Mysteries," with full color close-ups of ravaged skin and the victims' personal accounts. In spring 2006, the CDC acknowledged the "volume of concern" about the syndrome and last summer established an online contact for fearful victims.

The agency has since received about 1,200 inquiries, and is intent on providing "meaningful answers." said Dr. Pearson.

Over the next year, the CDC will track Morgellons patients in California who have reported symptoms in the past eighteen months using Kaiser Permanente facilities in Oakland.

On January 17, 2008, the CDC reported they will bring in military to investigate the condition known as Morgellons.

On January 25th, 2008, a petition was circulated to request the CDC to investigate this phenomenon by the Morgellons Research Foundation:

The undersigned citizens of the United States urgently request a

U.S. government oversight hearing to determine why the Centers for Disease Control (CDC) are taking so long to investigate the cause of Morgellons disease. The CDC has admitted that it has been receiving citizen complaints of symptoms of this disease for over a decade. Letters from senators from a number of states to the CDC calling for action on this apparently infectious condition that now affects about 9,000 families have resulted in NO apparent investigation thus far by the CDC. Recently, a government oversight hearing was called for to investigate complaints of contaminated pet food and determined that there was system wide failure by the FDA to protect pets from contaminated foods. We believe ill and suffering individuals are at least as important as sick pets. There were a number of pet deaths attributable to tainted pet food. At least 15 persons have died directly or indirectly after being affected by Morgellons disease and thousands more are suffering and becoming disabled.

Most were misdiagnosed as being delusional by dermatologists, largely untrained in psychiatric conditions, using badly flawed inaccurate and unsupportable assertions in the literature. Scientists have identified some of the physical manifestations of this disease using dermatoscopes, microscopes, DNA analysis and chromatography. The manifestations of this disease are real, multisystem and progressive, not delusional. However the etiologic agent has so far not matched any known human pathogen. There is no cure. Time is of the essence since one half of the 9000 people identifying themselves as ill with this disease have done so within the past six months. This may represent an emerging epidemic. In our opinion, the CDC is failing in its obligation of "controlling the introduction and spread of infectious diseases," and we, the taxpayers have a right to know why this is happening and to have the current apparent failure of the CDC addressed immediately.

I signed my name to this petition added a footnote that I would be agreeable to a call and left my phone number. I sent it to: Centers for Disease Control and Prevention, 1600 Clifton Rd, Atlanta, GA 30333, U.S.A. Switchboard: (404) 639-3311 / Public Inquiries: (404) 639-3534/ (800) 311-3435. I did receive an acknowledgement but have never received any other inquiry regarding any details of my own illness.

I decided to also contact my U.S. Senator from Minnesota Norm

Coleman on January 27, 2008.

Dear Senator Coleman,

I just recently discovered that the CDC has announced that they would formally investigate the disease known as Morgellons syndrome. I am totally in favor of us directing resources to find the cause and possibly the cure.

From 1996 to 2001 I battled this disease or something similar. It is the most baffling awful disease anyone can have and totally misunderstood by our medical establishment. I turned to natural methods to find relief and have it under control.

It is entirely possible that the suspect nematodes that can cause this disease are the basis for other debilitating illnesses . . . like chronic fatigue, fibromyalgia, and other auto-immune diseases. We could easily be at the tip of the ice-berg in numbers of cases and unless we direct resources we could be caught with an out of control infectious disease much worse than Aids.

Sincerely yours,
Karen Ament

Reply written on February 11, 2008
From: Coleman.senate.gov

Dear Mrs. Ament,

Thank you for taking the time to contact Senator Coleman regarding Morgellons Syndrome. We appreciate your sharing how this disease has personally impacted you and support efforts to help understand, present, and treat this disease.

As you know, the CDC recently announced it would begin studying this disease with the help of the U.S. Armed Forces Institute of Pathology as well as the American Academy of Dermatology. Since this investigation is still in its beginning stages, findings and recommendations have not yet been released. However, please know that we will continue to monitor this issue closely with your story and thoughtful advice in mind.

Thank you once again for contacting us and please do not hesitate to contact us on any issue of concern to you and your family.

Sincerely, Senator Norm Coleman - Minnesota

Even before the study results were released, Morgellon activists were certain that the CDC was not taking this disease seriously. Cliff Mickelson – (I have permission to reprint)

Much sound and fury is currently being generated by mainstream media concerning the recent CDC announcement that Kaiser Permanente has been selected by the CDC to conduct a "groundbreaking" study into the causes and nature of what the CDC and Kaiser both euphemistically (and erroneously) term Morgellons "syndrome."

In the opening news conference statement to the press, the CDC's principle investigator Dr. Michele Pearson, with his Kaiser counterpart, Dr. Joe Selby at his side, sets the tone for a CDC position on this issue that can only be described as disingenuous at best.

"There is insufficient information," intones Dr. Pearson, "to determine whether persons who identify themselves as having this condition, have common cause for their symptoms or may share common risk factors."

This statement speaks volumes. One can only suppose that the good doctor is under-informed.

The CDC is quite clearly aware that there already exists a large body of professional Morgellons research that has been done under the organized auspices of former Morgellons research Foundation scientist Dr. Randy Wymore.

Dr. Wymore, the current head of Morgellons research at the prestigious school of Pharmacology at Oklahoma State University, has personally briefed CDC officials in the past. Nonetheless, the Atlanta based organization showed very little interest in the subject of Morgellons, or in Dr. Wymore's revolutionary findings concerning the growing danger this affliction poses to society at large.

The CDC is also aware that there exists a large compendium of additional work available for referencing. A great deal of research has been performed in the last few years by a select number of other professionally qualified medical-field researchers including such well known notables as Dr. William Harvey, Dr. Hildegard Stannigar, and Dr. Rahim Karjoo.

In his opening CDC press conference statement Dr. Pearson uses the term "common risk factors" as a descriptive term . . . For those who are the uninitiated that is CDC doublespeak for drug abuse or delusional mental illness.

This denigrating and underhanded remark is a direct slap in the face of Morgellons patients, many of whom are children, senior citizens, teachers, nurses, or other medical professionals.

For reasons they have apparently chosen not to make public, the CDC has, therefore, deliberately decided to ignore, negate and suppress the considerable body of nearly three years' worth of ongoing, highly qualified field work by others outside the CDC nexus.

By marginalizing professional research that has already taken place during the CDC's long and curious absence from the Morgellons issue, they now seem to be suddenly setting themselves up as the sole judge of any consequence in the public eye.

Is this cynical lip service designed to throw a fog over the clever methodology of how bureaucracies with something to hide engage in issue assassination?

Why would they spend hard-earned tax dollars for information that already exists and could be had with a simple conference call or two? Well, the answer is at once simple and yet Byzantine.

It is germane to note that by their own admission, over the last eight years the CDC has received thousands upon thousands of requests for help from Morgellons victims. All of these pleas, until now, fell upon deaf ears. No money was ever spent to determine what it was that was taking place not only across America but around the world as well. Meanwhile the CDC has spent millions of taxpayer dollars on an unending parade of fizzled "non-event" epidemics that have come and gone during that same time frame. A number of these high-dollar non-event epidemics affected less than a dozen people across the country while others never materialized at all!

As the white rabbit would say: Curiouser and curiouser! A pitiful three hundred and sixty thousand dollars is all that is earmarked for this study! What will three hundred and sixty thousand dollars buy in today's world of bloated research budgets? The salaries of the research staff alone should total more than that. What can we assume will be the cost of high technology tests and other high-tech equipment needed to insure accurate Morgellons test results? Modern research tests can easily run into the hundreds of thousands of dollars. Private researcher Dr. Hildegaard Stannigar reports that she has independently spent thirty-nine thousand dollars of private money on such tests and that many more tests are still in need of performing.

It doesn't take an accountant to figure out that three hundred and sixty thousand dollars is not going to buy much in the way of a reliable study—and—it doesn't take a weatherman to figure out which way the wind is blowing in the halls of the CDC.

Morgellons activists need to wake up and smell the coffee. The

CDC has no intention of solving the Morgellons mystery. Those who think otherwise need to review the history of the CDC's hostile and dismissive interaction with the Morgellons community over the span of the last eight to ten years. Under modest scrutiny it becomes painfully apparent that this study is a farce and a fraud.

What is actually being sold to the gullible among us is smoke and mirrors' for a variety of hidden reasons the CDC is offering up the public expedient of having done their "part."
Cliff Mickelson

On June 8th, 2012, I wrote to Cliff Mickelson.

Dear Cliff,

I was able to access your web site last p.m. "Groundbreaking Morgellons Study a Fraud," and thoroughly enjoyed it.

You confirmed my very thoughts.

In 1996 I contracted a disease very similar to Morgellons and fought it for a five-year period. I still need to do maintenance, but I am well now. Early on I contacted Mary Leito and Randy Wymore and others in the forefront of investigating this disease. I told Mary I was planning on writing a book, but, as of this date, I have not finished it. My manuscript is getting close to finishing though.

I would like to ask your permission to include your data on the CDC/Kaiser "Ground Breaking Morgellons Study a Fraud," if I could? In the last chapters of my book I am addressing this very same issue. I myself had early contact with the CDC and my senator at the time contacted them on my behalf but twelve years later they have yet to contact me ever.

Thank you so much for consideration of my request.

Sincerely,
Karen Ament

In the throes of my illness, I would have gladly accepted any prescription to actually cure my malady but a psychosomatic diagnosis and subsequent prescribing of psychotropic medicines would have not done a single thing to alleviate the dermatological symptoms I was having. The drugs would most certainly have put me in a reduced state of awareness and calmed my fears and made me into a complacent patient. I would have none of that and just wanted to be rid of the doggone thing, which I knew was real and raging within my body.

It seems that the CDC spending a miserable three hundred and sixty thousand dollars to six hundred thousand dollars (depending on sources quoted) for the touted study, would be ashamed of themselves for actually saying that their study was the end all and be all of the debate.

The old adage can be used here—put your money where your mouth is. The CDC has done just that with the amount of money spent on their Unexplained Dermopathy Study.

Is it possible that by barely spending a pittance to catch a possibly dangerous disease that could have come out of a bioterror lab, the CDC will have to face a major onslaught down the road to the consternation of our entire country or even the world? Hindsight will give us the answer but the poor suffering people are pleading for an answer now. Logic will tell anyone looking into Morgellons that studies about the incubation periods by the sufferers are very short . . . many in several hours to several days. How in the world does that translate into mental illness in any way, shape, or form? These people were highly functioning individuals until the minute or hour they somehow contracted this THING! Do your homework, doctors, and ask questions about the past history of these patients and keep in mind it is nearly impossible to develop a full blown mental illness in a few hours or a few days.

Chapter Eighteen

Ongoing Research
& Communication

T HIS IS THE LETTER I WROTE to Dr. Randy Wymore after perusing his position statement on the Topic of Morgellons Disease and other Morgellons related issues written on June 19th, 2007.

1/27/2008
To: Morgellons @OKState.EDU
Subject: Thank you!
Dear Dr. Wymore,

After contracting what appears to be similar to Morgellons in 1996 I was amazed to tune in to all the attention this bizarre affliction has been receiving. I thought I was the only one who had it.

I kept carefully documented notes (registered nurse background) and am mostly well now. I turned to natural anti-parasitic routines to rid myself of the disgusting symptoms.

My heart breaks that there are so many others who are just now trying to deal with their symptoms. It is both surreal and yet so obvious with the physical manifestations ever present.

I am concerned that we are entering an era of an infectious disease that knows no barriers and will be very difficult if not impossible for our medical community to treat. They cannot look beyond established pharmaceutical treatments that simply will not work for very few of Morgellons symptoms.

We need researchers like you to think outside of the box.

If I can be of any help in giving background etc. please contact me.

Thank you very much.

Sincerely,
Karen Ament

I also wrote to Mary Leitao, the discoverer of today's Morgellons Disease.

January 29, 2008
Morgellons Research Foundation
PO Box 357
Guilderland, N.Y.
c/o Mary M. Leitao

Dear Mary,

We subscribe to the *Washington Times* and an article caught my eye entitled, "CDC enlists military to study mysterious, frightening skin ailment," in the January 21, 2008, edition. I could hardly believe what I was reading because in July of 1996 I contracted a mysterious disease very similar to Morgellons. It took me many years to again be fully functioning. I am a trained registered nurse and have always been a note taker. Needless to say I filled many notebooks that outline my progression from total bewilderment to raw determination to despair and then back and forth many many times. This was a doozy unlike anything I could have ever imagined. I feel I could possibly be of assistance to a researcher and am willing to do so. Because I am now in remission (with just a few symptoms now and then) some of my remedies could be interesting to sufferers. I was open to anything when I realized that the medical community (many who were our friends) could not help me. I searched out of the box, which at first felt so strange as I was not taught that this was permissible. I was just so determined that this thing was not going to kill me; there had to be a God-given remedy somewhere. I used products available from health food stores and Hanna's Herb shop in Colorado. Considering my successful outcome the cost was minimal.

If I can be of any assistance to you, your family, or others please let me know. I would be happy to write up a summary based on my notes. I always thought I would write a book and now may be the time with the renewed interest in Morgellons.

Please know there is a cure or at least a remission; I am living proof. My severe arthritis symptoms even went away.

My best to you and your suffering family.

Sincerely,
Karen Ament
P.S. copy to Randy S. Wymore, Ph.D.

Mary answered my letter.

From: Mary Leitao
Executive Director
Morgellons Research Foundation
Subject: Morgellons
Thursday, 31 January 2008

Dear Karen,

We received your registration. If you would like to be called by a member of our board of directors who lives in Minnesota, please email your phone number to me. Are you an R.N.?
Love,
Mary

From: Karen Ament
To: Morgellons Mary Leitao
Date: Thursday, 31 January 2008

Dear Mary,

It is a pleasure to hear from you. I am so very sorry about the sad journey you and your family have made working through the awful details of this bizarre disease. I really thought I was the only one that had this disease and actually I wish I could still feel that way. My heart just breaks that so many people are at the end of their ropes and especially the little children.

Now that I am well I have tried to put this totally out of my mind and am not anxious to bring back all the horrible details - BUT - my love for my fellow man just cannot permit me to sweep it under a rug. If I can help in any way I must do so.

Yes, I am an R.N. but have not been active as my husband and I started a business in 1971 that I was a partner in. It would be fine if a Minnesota member of your board of directors calls me. They can call me at our home number.

You and your family will be in my prayers.

Sincerely,
Karen

On February 5, 2008, I received this letter:

Karen,

I am a volunteer who oversees the P.O. Box in Guilderland and am authorized to open all mail received there. Your check has been deposited to the MRF fund, and the foundation has been notified of your donation. Thank you. I will be forwarding your letter to Mary Leitao.

I found your letter very interesting. The Morgellons research foundation, a non-profit agency, was formed by Mary Leitao and the Board of Directors primarily to raise awareness in the community of the prevalence of this emerging, bizarre condition and to raise funding for private research. If you have a chance to peruse the Morgellons.org website, you will see it took several years to convince the CDC to investigate this problem. They kept insisting it was a psychological problem. But the MRF encouraged people to write, fax, and call their congressional representatives and governors and people in the CDC and in infectious health agencies. It took thousands of communiques and a great deal of pressure from congress people for them to finally initiate a study at Kaiser in northern California. The study was given a wide press coverage by the CDC a few weeks ago, which is great. It makes the community more aware of something most people and doctors have never encountered (fortunately), and many people with the problem are relieved to find out they are not "crazy" and there is a name for what they have been suffering.

I did not know that the CDC had enlisted the military to study this skin ailment. As you know, it is not just a skin ailment; it can affect many parts of the body.

Private research is necessary because even though the CDC has finally been prevailed upon to study the matter (the study to be conducted by the very same doctors who have been denying its existence to their Morgellons patients at Kaiser). It will be a long time before they will be looking for a cause and a cure. But it is hoped they will validate the disease to stop the dermatologists in the United States from insisting that this is DOP.

Nonetheless, it is my personal opinion that alternative medicine is the way to go in this case. Drugs seem to help for a time, but things seem to get worse when one stops the drugs. I also think a good detox program is necessary and a strengthening of the immune system. I have this myself. I could really relate when you said "from total bewilderment to raw determination to despair and then back and forth many, many times.") Morgellons.org is not set up to suggest treatments to sufferers so I hope you will post your success in dealing with this condition to one or more of the support groups already set up on the internet. I am also personally interested in how you brought about your remission.

If you care to discuss it with me, please drop me a note at the P.O. Box and I will call you on the phone.

Cristina
MRF
P.O. Box 357
Guilderland, NY 12084-0357

Correspondence from Dr. Randy Wymore . . .
From: Morgellons MORGELLONS@OKSTATE.EDU
RE: Thank you!
Wednesday 30 January 2008

Please feel free to email anything you feel may help us in our research.
Thank you!
Jennifer Burkeen, BS
Research Assistant
Dept. of Pharmacology & Physiology
Oklahoma State University
Center for Health Sciences and College of Osteopathic Medicine
111 W. 17th Street, Tulsa, Oklahoma 74107
Author note: I continue to donate to Dr. Wymore's ongoing research in hopes his lab will find a breakthrough that so many are praying for.

From Mary Leitao
To: Morgellons @aol.com
Subject: Thank you Mary
Date: Sun, 10 Feb 2008

Dear Mary,

Greetings to you!

I want to thank you very much for asking R.H. to get in touch with me. We had a long conversation about the scourges of living with Morgellons and the cause and effect. It is unbelievable to hear his stories. Many people have literally lost everything.

After pondering the situation and my involvement as a sufferer myself (since 1996) I decided to write a book (albeit a small one). I am in touch with a publisher. I have started writing my manuscript.

I feel this would be a way for Morgellon sufferers to see the scope of what is happening in the way of research, things to do to alleviate their suffering, and to see so many others are dealing with the same or similar symptoms. It also would be good if their doctors could possibly read it so they would be taken more seriously.

I would very much like to include in my book testimonials. Would it be possible for you to contact Morgellon registrants and ask them if they would like to participate? It could be done on an anonymous basis.

Please let me know your ideas on my request.

I would really appreciate your assistance.

Thank you very much,

Sincerely,

Karen Ament

Authors note: My outline changed dramatically since I first had ideas to formulate a working hypothesis about this possible emerging disease, Morgellons. But all books are created with first an idea; the working outline can come much later. Because you are reading this, this is the later I hoped would come someday but the working outline does not include any patient follow-up by me. The scope of this disease has magnified to the degree that only a research lab can possibly handle the voluminous paper work that would result in assembling meaningful patient data.

To: Morgellons @aol.com
Subject: Re: Thank you Mary
Date: Sun, 10 Feb 2008
Dear Mary,

Thanks for your swift reply . . . I really appreciate it.

I can understand your reluctance considering that it might be upsetting to registrants.

All I would need is this data:

Year contracted, symptoms, treatment, if any, status now and submitted by: Initials only and the State they reside in.

There would be no interviews to upset them in any way. They could e-mail or mail the info to me. That way you would not have to be involved. I would be happy to share any data I receive with you if it would help you in any way with your research. Perhaps it could be handled by a notation on your web site that an author is seeking research information (see above) to help inform the public about the sufferers of Morgellons and offer suggestions as to how she was able to overcome this disease. My e-mail and address could be given out to anyone interested.

Thanks a lot Mary,
Sincerely,
Karen Ament

Author's note: Since this writing the Morgellons Research Foundation has been disbanded. Other organizations are assuming some of the vision, among them the Charles E. Holman Foundation and Dr. Randy Wymore's research being done at Oklahoma University

Reply from Mary . . .
Sunday, 10 February 2008
Subject: Re: Thank you Mary

Hi Karen,

We have been asked to help others write books over the years and although we did try to help connect people, this was not always well-received by registrants. I will discuss it with the board again, and will let you know if this seems like something we could do, since as I said we have tried this type of thing in the past but it didn't work out. Please let me know if there is anything else I can do.
Mary

From: Karen Ament
To: Cristina MRF
Date: Friday, 15 February 2008

Dear Cristina,

I so appreciated receiving your letter. I am so very sorry however that you have Morgellons. I have sent to you via snail mail copies of my rough draft for the book I am trying to write. Because I am in remission or possibly cured I feel I need to let as many people know as possible what I did to get there. Also because it was multifaceted I have to study my notes and try to determine what I took and when and my notes regarding the outcomes.

But until I get there I feel you and possibly others could see what I think the basics of treatment were for me. I totally agree with you that alternative medicine is the way to go. A good detox program is great but there is a proliferation of them on the market and it's hard to know which one to do. As you may know you will get worse before you get better. If the symptoms were too pronounced I stopped a bit, but got right back on as I knew it was working.

My program:

1. BLACK WALNUT

2. WORMWOOD

3. CLOVES (I added extra cloves and made my own in glycerin wrappers with blender blended whole cloves inside) I took two to three/day.

4. PAU d ARCO

When I started to treat in 1997 I had to find all these items on my own but now there is a very good kit that you can buy. It is Paragon by Renew Life; you can get it at most health food stores. I followed the kit information included as close as possible. I also did several fasts during my recovery.

I did the Paragon for 10 days and then did this for the 5 day rest and then another 10 days on Paragon.

1. Colloidal silver- (I now make my own) I also used a squirt bottle to squirt it into my nose.

2. Oregano oil- drops under tongue hold twenty seconds

3. Aloe vera

4. Fiber smart by Renew Life

I continued to do this regimen until these products were gone.

After the cleanse, I also took these items but not necessarily in this order:

1. Shark cartilage

2. L. Cysteine

3. Vitamin A

4. Red clover blossoms

5. Grape juice

6. Pumpkin seeds – eat them

7. Golden seal

8. Milk thistle

9. Licorice root

10. Acidophilus

11. St. John's Wort

12. Multi vitamin – a good one.

I also took these products so I could sleep (not at the same time however)

1. Melatonin
2. Ornithine
3. Valerian

I also did other things throughout my recovery but they are too numerous to go into here.

And Cristina don't forget to turn to our loving God for His mercy. On your knees pray as hard as you ever have. "BE STRONG AND OF GOOD COURAGE; BE NOT FRIGHTENED, NEITHER BE DISMAYED; FOR THE LORD YOUR GOD IS WITH YOU WHEREVER YOU GO." Josh. 1-9 (NIV)

God's blessings on you as you recover with His help.
Warm regards,
Karen
Ps It is okay to share this info but at this point please keep my name anonymous. Thank you.

Obviously I did not write my book for years after I planned to do so. Even though I've done it now, I feel deep regret that I didn't make it more of a priority in order to give hope and possibly even relief to many sufferers. And even more importantly light a fire under some medical professionals to PAY ATTENTION to not just what their patients are saying is happening now but their past history. These are real people many of them children that just logically cannot develop a full blown mental illness instantaneously.

Many health professionals continue to mistake Morgellons disease for a psychosomatic disorder, despite numerous laboratory and physical abnormalities including central nervous system, cardiac, pulmonary and kidney effects, and resetting of several autonomic and endocrine control loops.

The illness has been the subject of reports by major news outlets including Fox, CNN, NBC, ABC, NPR, *The Washington Post*, *People Magazine*, and *Newsweek* as well as local news outlets around the world since the Morgellons label first appeared in 2002. More than thirteen thousand families from all fifty states as well as forty-five nations have voluntarily registered their symptoms with the MRF, suggesting this number represents only a fraction of the true number of families affected by the illness.

Chapter Nineteen

The Charles E. Holman Morgellons Disease Foundation

O UR ORGANIZATION EXISTS to play an integral role in spreading the understanding of Morgellons disease to others." Charles "Chas" Holman (www.the cehf.org)

"The Charles E. Holman Foundation is a grassroots activist organization that supports research, education, diagnosis, and treatment of Morgellons Disease. Ultimately, we seek discovery of its cause and cure."

"In 2004 Charles and Cindy (Casey) Holman were determined to find answers about an unusual and debilitating condition, Morgellons disease (MD), which Cindy was dealing with. The New Morgellons Order was founded with strong commitments to honesty and integrity. The goals were and remain directed towards funding scientific research, promoting public awareness and educating the medical community through factual information with scientific merit. Officially receiving the status of 501© 3 non-profit in 2006, the organization's name was amended with the IRS in 2007 under 'doing business as' to include the Charles E. Holman Foundation to honor our founder for the work he had begun. Charles passed away in 2007 from heart related issues and did not have MD. Cindy Casey-Holman, R.N. serves as the director of the CEHF continuing to lead the fight for Morgellons patients everywhere."

The 10th Annual Medical-Scientific Conference on Morgellons Diseases and rally was held at the Capitol (April 29th to May lst, 2017) in Austin, Texas.

The Charles E. Holman Foundation and Morgellons Disease have been added to the data base of the Genetic and Rare Disease Information Center (GARP) and are the recognized "go-to" resource for M.D.

Chapter Twenty

MRF Disbanded

The current status as of the Morgellons Research Foundation as of June 2013, notification on the MRF website is:

The Morgellons Research Foundation is no longer an active organization and is not accepting registrations or donations.

The MRF donated its remaining funds to the Oklahoma State University Foundation to support their Morgellons disease research.

This came as a surprise to me as I had first contacted Mary Leitao the executive director of the Morgellons Research Foundation in 2008 and just assumed since there was still no discovery or cure that the Foundation would continue to operate until that was the case. I was happy to hear that they have expressed faith in work of Dr. Randy S. Wymore, who is the director of the ODU-CHS Center for the Investigation of Morgellons Disease at Oklahoma State University. Dr. Wymore is a regular speaker at the Charles E. Holman Foundation annual conference.

Because the MRF was in the forefront of research and discovery, it is important to include here their latest position paper printed before they disbanded.

The Morgellons Research Foundation (MRF) is a 501©3 non-profit organization established in 2002 in honor of a two-year-old child with an unknown illness, which his mother labeled "Morgellons disease." The MRF is dedicated to raising awareness and research funding for this poorly understood illness, which can be disfiguring and disabling, and affects people of all age groups including an increasing number of children. The number of families currently registered with the MRF is believed to represent a fraction of the true number of affected families.

The MRF fully supports the formal efforts by the CDC and Kaiser Permanente's Northern California Division of Research to investigate Morgellons disease. The MRF will continue to financially assist the ongoing efforts of private research scientists who are dedicated to solving the mystery of this tragic illness.

I would like to take this opportunity to thank Mary Leitao and her dedicated board members for their impressive service to mankind. Their efforts while not immediately successful will serve as the springboard and the catalyst for any future discoveries to solve this mysterious disease Morgellons. Please know that you will go down in the annals of history as unafraid to buck the system in place and are true pioneers.

"A journey of a thousand miles begins with a single step."
Lao-tzu, Chinese philosopher (604 B.C. to 531 B.C.)

Chapter Twenty-One

Mayo Clinic Study

A STUDY OF 108 PERSONS IDENTIFIED with delusional skin infestation, including persons with Morgellons, examined between 2001 and 2007 at the Mayo Clinic was published in *Archives of Dermatology* on May 16, 2011. "The study did not find evidence of skin infestation despite examination of specimens provided by the patients and study of skin biopsies of study participants. The authors concluded the study results were consistent with the participant's original diagnosis of delusional infestation. They reported that about two thirds of the skin biopsies showed dermatitis, and stated that the skin condition and resultant distress might play a role in the patient's delusional or 'false belief' their skin is infested by pathogens. Until a treatable infectious component is identified, patients can continue to be treated with neuroleptics- pimozide, risperidone, aripiprazole which have been reportedly effective."

Until this disease is labeled and correct treatments are advised to alleviate, this cat-and-mouse game will continue between patients and their doctors. When people know they have physical symptoms and can see and feel the turmoil in their bodies, they will have none of an explanation that does not address any of that. They say to themselves, I was functioning fine in all respects until I suddenly came down with THIS THING. It becomes very hard if not impossible to convince them that they now have a mental illness.

All one has to do is read the possible side effects of the three prescription medications that the Mayo Clinic recommends and one is taken aghast at what will happen to a percentage of people that are treated with these medications for Morgellons symptoms. They are assuming that the delusions will be able to be done away with by the use of these antipsychotics. But let's just think what will happen if the delusions go away but the symptoms do not and medication side effects will further compound the scenario. You now have a formerly high-functioning individual who could in all possibilities been treated in a responsible manner based on a good case history, chronological evidence gathering, charting on and treating the symptoms relegated to a life of living with and trying to treat all the side effects of the very medicines supposed to heal them in the first place. Plus, their original alarming symptoms are still there and getting worse by the hour and day.

Hopefully integrative medicine will be practiced by the doctors that these poor suffering Morgellons symptom patients see, and until a cure or discovery is found, they at least will not be made worse.

The Hippocratic Oath is an oath historically taken by physicians and other health care professionals swearing to practice medicine honestly. It is widely believed to have been written by Hippocrates, often regarded as the father of western medicine, or by one of his students.

HIPPOCRATIC OATH - MODERN VERSION

"I swear to fulfill, to the best of my ability and judgement, this covenant:

"I will respect the hard-won scientific gains of those physicians in whose steps I walk, and gladly share such knowledge as is mine with those who are to follow.

"I will apply, for the benefit of the sick, all measures (that) are required, avoiding those twin traps of overtreatment and therapeutic nihilism.

"I will remember that there is art to medicine as well as science, and that warmth, sympathy and understanding may outweigh the surgeon's knife or the chemist's drug.

"I will not be ashamed to say "I know not," nor will I fail to call in my colleagues when the skills of another are needed for a patient's recovery.

"I will respect the privacy of my patients, for their problems are not disclosed to me that the world may know. Most especially must I tread with care in matters of life and death. If it is given me to save a life, all thanks. But it may also be within my power to take a life; this awesome responsibility must be faced with great humbleness and awareness of my own frailty. Above all, I must not play at God.

"I will remember that I do not treat a fever chart, a cancerous growth, but a sick human being, whose illness may affect the person's family and economic stability. My responsibility includes these related problems, if I am to care adequately for the sick.

"I will remember that I remain a member of society, with special obligations to all my fellow human beings, those of sound of mind and body as well as the infirm.

"If I do not violate this oath, may I enjoy life and art, respected while I live and remembered with affection thereafter. May I always act so as to preserve the finest traditions of my calling and may I long experience the joy of healing those who seek my help."

This was written in 1964 by Louis Lasagna, Academic Dean of the School of Medicine at Tufts University , and used in many medical schools today.

After reading the Mayo Clinic study reported in 2011, I thought about how close I was to go to the Mayo Clinic if the University of Minnesota was not able to diagnose me! The University of Minnesota was not able to diagnose me and thankfully I chose not to go to Mayo. Instinctively I felt state-of-the-art beliefs regarding this perplexing illness would continue. After reading about their study done between 2001 and 2007, I knew Mayo had no answers. When I thought of the thousands and thousands of suffering people with a disease that remains undiagnosed but in the meantime is classified as delusions of parisitosis by one of the foremost medical teaching hospitals in the world; I must somehow find the time to keep writing.

After all, I am now a seventy-six-year-old grandmother that should be baking cookies, playing golf or caring for and enjoying her grandchildren.

What in the world am I doing facing off against the elite medical researchers at the Mayo Clinic? I could not hold a candle to any of the educated researchers. All I have is a life story to tell that is bizarre and frustrating but with a happy ending (but only for me). So many others that relied on our medical system had no hope at all especially after this report was published by the Mayo Clinic. Where is the hope for a cure? At least I had that when I turned to naturopathic remedies. I could feel the changes taking place for the better with each remedy I tried. I knew I was on the right track. When I did consult doctors, I no longer asked them anything about the fight of my life (I was on my own for that). I only asked them about managing my subsidiary diagnoses . . . eye disease, hypothyroidism, atrial fibrillation, polymyalgia, and giant cell arteritis and now cancer. I never discussed my ongoing battle with my new doctors. Why destroy our relationship? I did not have to drag them into this thing of mine. They are wonderful listeners and caring doctors.

I became sure that God has a unique sense of humor. Why me, Lord, came to mind more than once. Why couldn't I have gotten something that ended in a dramatic fashion with doctors cheering my recovery? Instead I recovered from something they never knew I had.

After all this twenty-first-century modern medicine is unarguably the state of the art. But if we can't test for it, it doesn't exist.

Somehow I was spared from going down that long road of non-recovery. I am so thankful for my dear Lord that He gave me the strength and determination to think outside of the box. Perhaps even I could help others with a retelling of my tale of woe!

Would this account possibly stir a researcher or scientific doctor to step outside the box as well and put their brains to work to put this medical puzzle together? After all medical miracles are taking place in so many fields. I remember seeing one of the first open heart surgeries at my county hospital, Ancker Hospital in St. Paul, Minnesota. We student nurses felt such a privilege to even be in the same room with these pioneers. Why can't this same can-do spirit prevail now? Why can't our medical people unleash the energy of discovery of an impossible new illness and then a cure? Have we become so entrenched with the pharmaceutical industry calling all the shots? Or is it something else entirely? Why is it if there isn't a diagnosis for something, it simply can't exist?

End of the Story
or
IS IT JUST THE BEGINNING OF THE STORY?

Addendum

Morgellons Research Time Line

2002 - Mary Leitoa identified disease and started the Morgellons Research Foundation (informally) .

2002 - Mary Leitoa named her son's illness Morgellons.

2003 - June - Letter from Stan Husted, MDH and MPA Supervising Heath, Biolgist C.A. Liforni, Department of Health Services Vector-Borne Disease Section to Mary Leito Regarding California residents that have contracted her Morgellons Symptoms and concerns.

2003 - October - Letter from Stan Husted regarding contact with the J.S. Centers for Disease Control and Prevention (COC). Advice is to stand by June 2003 letter.

2004 - Mary Leitoa founded the Morgellons Research Foundation as a non profit.

2004 - Mary Leitoa put up web site Morgellons Research Foundation.

2004 - Charles & Cindy (Casey) Holman founded the New Morgellons Order.

2006 - August - 2006 V27 i 18 pl (2) Dermatology Times, Bill Gillette - Staff correspondent CoC to Investigate Mysteries of Morgellons Disease (News) Clinical Report.

2006 – August - Morgellons featured in a "Medical Mysteries" segment on ABC's *Prime Time Live*.

2006 – October – CDC sends Morgellons investigators to California. Bill Gillette. *Dermatology Times.*

2006 - CDC task force consisting of 12 people formed.

2006 – CDC implemented a Morgellons information and voicemail line at (404) 718-1199, which people who believe they may have the disease can call for help.

2006 - Charles E. Holman Foundation founded.

2006 - November 1 - Dr. Gregory V. Smith M.D., IAAP, NMO letter. Tips on Surviving Your Doctor Appointment.

2007 - Charles & Cindy (Casey) Holman changed the status to a non-profit . . . Charles E. Holman Foundation.

2007 - 8,000 people had responded to Mary Leitoa's Morgellons Research Foundation website.
June 19th - Dr. Randy Wymore, Ph. D., released position statement on Morgellons disease.

2007 - June 21st - *The Washington Times* by Jennifer Harper CDC Enlists Military to Study mysterious Frightening Skin Ailment.

2007 - August - CDC issued statement "Morgellons Is an Unexplained and Debilitating Condition That Has Emerged as a Publlic Health Concern.

2007 - November - CDC announced investigation under way (website up . . . Unexplained Dermopathy).

2007- June 19 - Dr. Randy Wymore, Ph.D. released position statement on Morgellons disease.

2007 - June 21 - *The Washington Times* by Jennifer Harper CDC enlists military to study mysterious, frightening skin ailment.

2008 - First Medical Conference sponsored by CEHF - Continues to present time.

2008 - January 25 - Petition circulated to request the CDC to investigate by the Morgellons Research Foundation.

2008 – February 11 – Mn Senator Norm Coleman reply – "CDC recently announced it will begin studying this disease with the help of the U.S. Armed Forces Institute of Pathology as well as the American Academy of Dermatology."

2008 - June 17 - CDC enlisted aid of U.S. Armed Forces.

2009 – July 1 – Morgellons disease, illuminating an undefined illness: a case series William T Harvey, Robert C Bransfield, Dana E. Mercer, Andrew J Wright, Rebecca M Ricchi and Mary M Leitao.

2009 - November 4 - CDC issued preliminary report.

2010 - Morgellons disease - Analysis of a population with clinically confirmed microscopic subcutaneous fibers of unknown etiology. Virginia Savely & Raphael B Stricker.

2010 - March 17 - Letter to Colleagues by Dr. Gregory V. Smith.

2010 - June 15th - CDC Morgellons Investigation "A Failure" Dr. Joe Sellog, Research Director for Kaiser Hospital in Oakland.

2010 - Archives of Dermatology by Sara A. Hylwa, et al, entitled "Delusional Infestation, Including Delusions of Parasitosis: Results of Histologic Examination of Skin Biopsy and patient provided skin specimens" Co-author Mark, D.P. Davis, M.D., Mayo Clinic.

2010 - November 7 - Report http://www.mayo clinic.com/health/morgellonsdisease - "Morgellons Disease: Managing a Mysterious Skin Condition."

2011 - March 24 - CDC completed data analysis.

2011 - October 29 - Morgellons Disease, Another Tick borne Co-Infection? Ginger Savely, DNP, FNP Has treated about 400 of these patients in her practice and she has four published peer reviewed articles on the topic of Morgellons disease.

2011 - November 14 - Filament formation associated with spirochetal infection: a comparative approach to Morgellons disease. Marianne J. Middelveen and Raphael B Stricker. And why this new study is so very important.

2012 - January 25 - CDC released results of study indicating that there were - no disease organisms present in people with Morgellons, the fibers consisted mainly of cellulose which suggested were likely cotton, and concluded that, in these respects, the condition was similar to commonly recognized conditions such as "delusional infestation."

2012 - February - Cliff Mickelson paper- CDC/Kaiser- Ground breaking "Morgellons" Study a Fraud.

2012 - March 6 - *Journal of Clinical and Experimental Dermatology Re-*

search article: "Morgellons disease: A Chemical and Light Microscopic Study" by Marianne J. Middelveen, Elizabeth H. Rasmussen, Douglas G. Kahn & Raphael B. Stricker.

2012 - June - Morgellons Study cited by faculty of 1000- (F1000) - Top two percent published. Article entitled: "Morgellons Disease: A Chemical and Light Microscopic Study" by Marianne J. Middelveen, Elizabeth H. Rasmussen, Douglas G. Kahn & Raphael B. Stricker. Published in the *Journal of Clinical & Experimental Dermatology Research*. (*See* Appendix: Recommended Reading, Resources, Organization.)

2012 - August 18 - Dr. Mark Eberhard CDC director of the Division of Parasitic Disease and Malaria (DPDM) Center for the Disease Control (CDC) Center for Global Health (CGH) regarding Morgellons Study - "However, the case is closed for the CDC at the moment, that's all I can say about it now."

2012 - November 2 - Marianne J. Middelveen. "Morgellons Disease & Bovine Digital Dermatitus."

2013 - January - The Characterization & Evolution of Dermal Filaments from Patients with Morgellons Disease - Marianne J. Middelveen, Peter M. Mayne, Douglas Kahn & Raphael Stricker.

2013 - January 28 - Association of Spirochetal Infection with Morgellon's Disease. Naruabbe J. Middelveen, Divya Burugu, Akhila Poruri, Jennie Burke, Peter J. Mayne, Eva Sapi, Douglas G. Kahn & Raphael B. Stricker.

2013 - Peter Mayne M.D., principal author - co-authors: Dr. John English, Dr. Edward Kilbane, Jennie Burke, Marianne J. Middelveen & Dr. Raphael Stricker - "Morgellons: a novel, dermatological perspective as the multisystem infective disease borreliosis."

2013 – Notification on the MRF website is. "The Morgelons Research Foundation is no longer an active organization and is not accepting registrations or donations. The MRF donated remaining funds to the Oklahoma State University Foundation to support this Morgellons disease research."

2013 - July 13 - NIH (National Institute of Health) lists Morgellons as rare disease.
http://www.rarediseases.info.nih.gov/gard/browse-by-first-letter/m

2013 - December 9 - The CEHF announced that they will team up with Dr. Eva Sapi for research at the University of New Haven. "The investigation of an infectious cause of Morgellons Disease: resulting data & information may bring validation to patients & help with the proper diagnosis and treatment of this disease." Dr. Eva Sapi, Ph.D.

2013 - Reprinted by Charles E. Holman Foundation - Author - Harry Quinn Schone - Examination of the power structures Between Morgellons Patients and the Medical Community.

2016 - March 31 Learning from Morgellons. Work in Progress Seminar. Harry Quinn Schone. History and Philosophy of Science, Department of Science and Technology Studies. University College, London, England. "Morgellons may or may not be a modern affliction, but the circumstances in which it exists are distinctly specific to the twenty-first century."
June 15 - Charles E. Holman Morgellons Disease Foundation Press Release, "Studies show that infections not delusion cause Morgellons Disease."

2017 - April 29 to May 1 - 10th Annual Medical Scientific Conference on Morgellons Disease in Austin, Texas.

2018 - February 12 onward. London Ancient Science Conference. Harry Quinn Schone. "We connect journalists to expert academics and promote UCL Research and teaching throughout the global media."
March 5 Austin, Texas. Charles E. Holman Morgellons Disease Foundation announces a new study that shows Morgellons disease is not a delusion. Review of Medical Literature exposes flaws in delusional description. "History of Morgellons Disease: From Delusion to Definition" written by microbiologist Marianne

Middleveen from Calgary, Canada, together with nurse practitioner Melissa Fesler and internist Raphael Stricker, M.D., from Union Square Medical Associates in San Francisco, California.

2018 - April 14th and 15th - 11th Annual Medical-Scientific Conference on Morgellon Disease in Austin, Texas.

2018 - April 30 - "Clinical Evaluation of Morgellon's Disease in a Cohort of North American Patients" by Melissa Feslert, Raphael Stricker, and Marianne Middelveen.

"It is time we acknowledge the evidence. Morgellon's disease is not a deliusional illness, but a dermatologic condition associated with Lyme disease." - Cindy Casey-Holman, director of the Charles E. Holman Morgellon's Disease Foundation (CEHMDF) of Austin, Texas. www.morgellonsdisease.com

Coming soon...A new film directed by Pi Ware, Emmy award-winning editor, *Skin Deep: The Battle Over Morgellons.* www.morgellonsmovie.org Iron Will Films LLC.

Note: This time line is not complete but gives a rough outline of the progress made to search for and find a cure for the Disease of the Century.

Tune in for the REST OF THE STORY...

Epilogue

Moving Forward

L
OOKING THROUGH THE PRISM of my earlier medical training as a registered nurse, I looked with disbelief on the malady, very similar to today's Morgellons, abruptly starting in 1996. I wondered how any of this could be (based on my medical training to follow doctor orders explicitly)? Doctors are trained to react unemotionally to a patient's symptoms so they can evaluate based on established criteria. The established criteria are state of the art. When a patient does not logically fit into the puzzle, they are trained to find the most pieces that do fit.

With Morgellons patients, very little seems to fit established protocols. But in the absence of any clinical data (blood, urine, stool and skin analysis) the doctors fall back to their first observation of the patient's description of seeing and feeling something moving on or under their skin. What else can this be? Delusional parasitology?

I am not sure how a person feels when they are delusional. Perhaps one fades in and out of logic, and this would apply to many aspects of their lives. Just taking a guess, but one has to question why the delusional person would choose to focus just on one aspect like parasites. One would think that there would be a multitude of circumstances that they could and would be delusional about? The fact that Morgellons patient's are all determined to be delusional about one very, very narrow scope and not about anything else in their lives should be a subject of question. Also the very real physical symptoms and real illness symptoms that follow the beginning of Morgellons should be taken into account. Why do these Morgellons patients start abruptly with skin sensation symptoms and then transgress into a multitude of physical symptoms like eye problems, thyroid function, heart problems, arthritis, joint pain,

149

intestinal problems, cancer, and auto-immune diseases?

Why do so many people (approximately 15,000 at this time and some Morgellons experts' say it may be one million worldwide) exhibit the almost identical symptoms in the very same clinical progression? More questions than answers.

I would have loved to bask in my being normal again after my cure and the intensive fight for my life. But how can I turn my back on so many suffering people who are in the middle of their nightmare? Their symptoms are as real as mine were. I know that if they don't find help soon, many of these chronic sufferers would develop major medical diagnoses and illnesses or worse. Being so sick with the obvious wasting of their bodies due to an organism taking over that was not supposed to be there is extremely difficult for people to handle no matter how strong they are. You instinctively *know* that the doctors are wrong and you are right . . . you have something dreadful and unconscionable and unmentionable. You develop anger and depression. Some even lose their spouses and jobs and homes. There are no support groups, no sympathy or empathy or treatment by caregivers. There is little if any discussion about it with family and friends due to their being unable to believe you in most instances. How could you start telling about something that is impossible?

It's a very lonely place to be. It is a desert. Without God and His Book and my Church and Bible study group and constant prayer, I am not sure if I could have moved through the first intense stages of my illness with the strength to fight to find a cure.

I prayed this prayer daily and found much strength in it.

JESUS, I am confident of your great and personal love for me revealed through the tenderness of your Sacred Heart. From this source of all goodness and mercy pour out upon me and all those dear to me every needed grace and blessing. In every difficulty I will immediately turn to you, knowing that you CARE, are most powerful to help and want only to draw us closer to our Heavenly Father.

SACRED HEART OF JESUS, I PLACE ALL MY TRUST IN YOU!

Understandably, Bob was having hard time dealing with my symptoms as well, but he was a rock during it all. He treated me as if I was normal, and we continued our normal life - for better or worse comes to mind. My health struggle brought on the worse, but fighting it with Bob's help and support brought on the better. Most nights I was awake more than I slept. It was just too distracting to be quiet as the itching and crawling and drilling pain became unbearable at night. It was better to get up and sit and read and ponder and pray.

Days were better, but when I became obsessed with finding a cure, our lives were taken over by this nightmare. I tried hard to strike a balance, but I can't say I attained that goal all the time.

The powers that be have spoken. They (CDC) have issued their final edicts, but their tiny funded study has proved nothing. They say the case is closed. But far from it so many of us say in unison and the audible vibrations are getting louder and louder. People are continuing to suffer with this strange malady and in increasing numbers. Eventually some entity will have to address this issue again and this time to do it with a sense of urgency and funds and the will to actually get to the bottom of this emerging unexplained illness.

I hope through reading this book sufferers will see that they can escape the living hell they find themselves in and become normal again. God helps those who help themselves. I hope they all will be able to say the words I can happily say now . . .

I FEEL NORMAL. THANK GOD FOR NORMAL.
AND I DID IT WITHOUT A DIAGNOSIS.

Appendix

Recommended Reading and Resources

1. *PDR for Herbal Medicines*. First Edition. The Information Standard for Complementary Medicine. Medical Economics Company. Montvale, New Jersey.
2. *Life Extension Disease Prevention and Treatment*. Expanded Fourth Edition. Disease Prevention and Treatment. P.O. Box 229120. Hollywood, Florida 33022-9120.
3. *Prescription for Nutritional Healing*. Second Edition. Penguin Group (USA). James F. Balch, M.D. & Phyllis A. Balch, C.N.C.
4. *The Herbal Drugstore*. Linda B. White, M.D., Steven Foster and the Staff of Herbs for Health. Rodale Inc.
5. *Foods That Heal*. Maureen Salaman. James F. Scheer. M.K.S. Inc. "Prevent or reverse more than 100 common ailments with the information in this book."
6. *Everybody's Guide to Homeopathic Medicines. Safe and Effective Remedies for You and Your Family*. Stephen Cumming, M. D., and Dana Ullman, M.P.H. 3rd Revised Edition. G.P. Putnam's & Sons New York.
7. *Spontaneous Healing*. Andrew Weil, M.D. Ballantine Books. Random House Inc. New York. "How to discover and enhance your body's natural ability to maintain and heal itself."
8. *The Cure for All Cancers*. Hulda Regehr Clark, P.H.D., N.D. New Century Press. U.S.A. "Including over 100 case histories of persons cured."
9. *The Cure for All Diseases*. Hulda Regehr Clark, P.H.D., N.D. New Century Press. U.S.A. "With many case histories."
10. *The Woman with a Worm in Her Head*. Pamela Nagami, M.D. St. Martin's Press. Renaissance Books. New York. "And other true stories of infectious disease."
11. *Traditional Herbals for Modern Living. Euro-American herbal wisdom for restoring your healthy balance*. Hanna Kroeger. Coyyright 1998 by Hanna's, Boulder, CO 80301 First Edition.
12. *Hanna's Herb Shop. Ageless Remedies from Mother's Kitchen*. Hanna Kroeger.
13. *Hanna's Herb Shop. Alzheimer's Science and God*. Hanna Kroeger.
14. *Hanna's Herb Shop. Arteriosclerosis and Herbal Chelation*. Hanna Kroeger.

15. *Hanna's Herb Shop. Free Your Body of Tumors and Cysts.* Hanna Kroeger.
16. *Hanna's Herb Shop. God Helps Those Who Help Themselves.* Hanna Kroeger.
17. *Hanna's Herb Shop. Good Health through Special Diets.* Hanna Kroeger.
18. *Hanna's Herb Shop. Help One Another, an Anthology of the Teachings and Remedies of Hanna Kroeger.* Hanna Kroeger.
19. *Hanna's Herb Shop. Instant Herbal Locator.* Hanna Kroeger.
20. *Hanna's Herb Shop. Instant Vitamin-Mineral Locator.* Hanna Kroeger.
21. *Hanna's Herb Shop. New Book on Healing.* Hanna Kroeger.
22. *Centering Prayer. Renewing an Ancient Christian Prayer Form.* M. Basil. Pennington, O.C.S.O.
23. *In Conversation with God. Daily Meditations Volume Two: Lent and Eastertide.*
24. *Do Whatever Love Requires.* Harriet Hammons & Carol Ameche.
25. *The Applause of Heaven.* Max Lucado.
26. *Journeys Home. A Coming Home Resource.* Marcus C. Grodi, M.Div.
27. *Jesus - The One and Only.* Beth Moore.
28. *The Web That Has No Weaver: Understanding Chinese Medicine.* Ted Kaptchuk.
29. *Meridians and Acupoints* (International Acupuncture Textbooks). Zhu Bing
30. Just Be Well. Thomas A. Sult M.D., RTC Publishing, Writers of the Rollins Tabbs Press, P.O. Box 511, Highland Park, Illinois, 60035, copyright 2013.

A Love Letter from God the Father

Father's Love Letter used by permission Father Heart Communications at 1999-2013 www.FathersLoveLetter.com.

A Love Letter from God the Father (Printed in its Entirety)

My Dear Child . . .

You may not know Me, but I know everything about you - Psalm 139:1

I know when you sit down and when you rise up - Psalm 139:2

I am familiar with all your ways - Psalm 139.3

Even the very hairs on your head are numbered - Matthew 10:29-31

For you were made in My image - Genesis 1:27

In Me you live and move and have your being - Acts 17:28

For you are My offspring - Acts 17:28

I knew you even before you were conceived - Jeremiah 1:4-5

I chose you when I planned creation - Ephesians 1: 11-12

You were not a mistake, for all your days are written in my book - Psalm 139:15-16

I determined the exact time of your birth and where you would live - Acts 17:26

You are fearfully and wonderfully made - Psalm 139:14

I knit you together in your mother's womb - Psalm 139:13

And brought you forth on the day you were born - Psalm 71:6

I have been misrepresented by those who don't know me - John 8: 41-44

I am not distant and angry but am the complete expression of love - 1 John 4:16

You see I've loved you from the beginning, long before you loved me - 1 John 4:19

And it is My desire to lavish my love on you - 1 John 3:1

Simply because you are my child and I am your Father - 1 John 3:1

I offer you more than your earthly father ever could - Matthew 7:11

For I am the perfect Father - Matthew 5:48

Every good gift that you receive comes from My hand - James 1:17

For I am your provider and I meet all your needs - Matthew 6:31-33

My plan for your future has always been filled with hope - Jeremiah 29:11

Because I love you with an everlasting love - Jeremiah 31:3

My thoughts toward you are countless as the sand on the seashore - Psalms 139:17-18

And I rejoice over you with singing - Zephariah 3:17

I will never stop doing good to you - Jeremiah 32:40

For you are My treasured possessions - Exodus 19:5

I desire to establish you with all My heart and all My soul - Jeremiah 32:41

And I want to show you great and marvelous things - Jeremiah 33:3

If you seek Me with all your heart, you will find Me - Deuteronomy 4:29

Delight in Me and I will give you the desires of your heart - Psalm 37.4

For it is I who gave you those desires - Philippians 2:13

I am able to do more for you than you could possibly imagine - Ephesians 3:20

For I am your greatest encourager - 2 Thessalonians 2:16-17

I am also the Father who comforts you in all your troubles - 2 Corinthians 1:3-4

When you are brokenhearted, I am close to you - Psalm 34:18

As a shepherd carries a lamb, I have carried you close to my heart - Isaiah 40:11

One day I will wipe away every tear from your eyes - Revelation 21:3-4

And I'll take away all the pain you have suffered on this earth - Revelation 21:3-4

I am your Father, and I love you even as I love my Son, Jesus - John 17:23

I love you so much I gave My one and only Son for you - John 3:16

For in Jesus, My love for you is revealed - John 17:26

He is the exact representation of My being - Hebrews 1:3

He came to demonstrate that I am for you, not against you - Romans 8:31

And He came to die in place of your sins - Romans 5:8

Jesus died so that you and I could be reconciled - 2 Corinthians 5:18-19

I am not counting your sins against you - 2 Corinthians 5:18-19

His death was the ultimate expression of My love for you - 1 John 4:10

I gave up everything I loved that I might gain your love - Romans 8:38-39

If you receive the gift of My Son Jesus, you receive Me - 1 John 2:23

And nothing will ever separate you from My love again - Romans 8:38-39

Come home and I'll throw the biggest party heaven has ever seen - Luke 15:7

I have always been Father, and will always be Father - Ephesians 3:14-15

My question is - Will you be my child? John 1:12-13
I am waiting for you - Luke 15:11-32

LOVE, YOUR DAD, ALMIGHTY GOD

Acknowledgements

The author deeply thanks Corinne Dwyer, Liz Dwyer, and Curtis Weinrich of North Star Press for their excellent assistance in the completion of this book. Your courtesy and exceptional professionalism is profoundly appreciated.
www.northstarpress.com

To our good health

Karen Ament

Karen Ament

CPSIA information can be obtained
at www.ICGtesting.com
Printed in the USA
LVHW011721180319
611006LV00007B/408